# The Field Analyzer Primer

## SECOND EDITION

edited by Mary Jean Haley

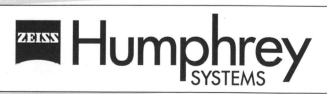
ZEISS Humphrey
SYSTEMS

San Leandro, California

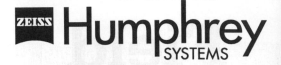

**3081 Teagarden Street
San Leandro, California 94577
510 895-9110
800 227-1508**

**Library of Congress Cataloging-in-Publication Data**

The Field analyzer primer.

Bibliography: p.
Includes index.
1. Perimetry—Technique.  2. Perimetry—Automation.
I. Haley, Mary Jean, 1945–        II. Allergan
Humphrey (Firm)
RE79.P4F54 1987        617.6'15        87–16900

ISBN 0-939-425-01-7

Printed in the United States of America
Third Printing, 1993

# Contents

# Illustrations

# Acknowledgments

**T**HIS *PRIMER* was written at the request of many practitioners who use the Humphrey Field Analyzer and is therefore dedicated to them.

In addition to this general encouragement, a number of people made important specific contributions to the Primer. For their generous help in our search for illustrative case histories we are indebted to Yvonne Alden; Roy W. Beck, MD; John A. Fleishman, MD; S. Samuel Gelbart, MD; Roger Gimbell, COA; the Glendale Eye Medical Group; George R. Hurd, OD; Marc F. Lieberman, MD; Christian Mageli, COA; V. Michael Patella, OD; Steven B. Perlmutter, MD; Linda Sexton, COT; and Scott D. Winjum, OD. Additional heartfelt thanks go to John A. Fleishman, MD and S. Samuel Gelbart, MD for their aid and advice on the preparation of sections on specific types of field defects. Anders Heijl, MD, Dunbar Hoskins, MD, Marc Lieberman, MD, Richard Mills, MD, and Jon A. Shiesel, MD kindly provided case histories for Statpac analysis. Thomas W. Raasch, OD was a great help with background research.

Allergan Humphrey staff members who deserve special thanks include V. Michael Patella, Allergan Humphrey's Director of Clinical Research, Chris Ritter, Director of Marketing, and Mee Mee Wong, Product Manager in charge of the Field Analyzer. Other Allergan Humphrey staff members who contributed were Jacki Chadwick and Ed Buliavac.

Preparation of the *Primer* has been in the general charge of Mary Jean Haley, who wrote much of the text and edited all of it.

The Allergan Corporation contributed invaluable financial support to this project.

# Introduction

# The Humphrey Field Analyzer Primer

**V**ISUAL FIELD testing gives the eye care practitioner essential information about the diagnosis and progress of major blindness-causing diseases. Field testing is, of course, a primary tool in diagnosing and monitoring glaucoma. Many other ocular and neurological diseases also produce characteristic patterns of field defects. Comprehensive visual field testing allows early detection and close monitoring of the progress of these diseases, enhancing the chances for successful treatment.

Although the usefulness of field testing has long been established, manual perimetry was a painstaking process that required the full attention of the doctor or a well-trained, experienced technician. Today, automated, computerized perimeters put very sensitive, highly precise perimetry within the reach of every practitioner. The tests do not have to be administered by a specialized technician, and the doctor's time and expertise are not needed until the test is completed and the results are ready for interpretation.

In addition to high test sensitivity and efficient use of clinic time, automated, computerized perimetry offers the doctor unprecedented flexibility. Visual field testing can now be tailored to the individual patient

1

and the individual practice. The doctor who specializes in the treatment of glaucoma, for example, can rely on the threshold testing strategies appropriate to the special demands of his or her practice. The practitioner with a more general patient population, on the other hand, will be able to offer patients field screening as a routine part of everyday practice.

Computerized perimetry offers a level of precision and a consistency of test method that were not generally possible with manual perimetry. The doctor can have confidence that in follow-up checks the test will be administered the same way each time, making test results genuinely comparable. The wide range of screening and thresholding tests and strategies available with the Humphrey Field Analyzer draws on the combined knowledge of the leading researchers in the field and incorporates the latest advances in visual field testing. Finally, with the Field Analyzer's Statpac program it is possible to perform an in-depth statistical analysis of test results at a speed and with a thoroughness that were simply out of reach of the everyday practitioner before computerization.

This *Primer* discusses Humphrey Field Analyzer software current in 1987. Earlier or later issues of Field Analyzer software may be slightly different. For a complete description of the Field Analyzer's features and operation, see the *Operator's Manual*. The *Statpac User's Guide* gives detailed directions for running Statpac analyses of test results.

# 1.

# Basic Principles of Perimetry

T HE NORMAL visual field extends more than 90°
temporally, 60° nasally and superiorly, and about
70° inferiorly. Most field testing initially concentrates
on the central 30°. Visual sensitivity is greatest in
the center, the fovea, and decreases toward the periphery. The field of vision is commonly represented as
the hill, or island, of vision (figure 1). The height and
shape of the normal hill of vision varies among
individuals with, to name just a few factors, age, the
general level of ambient light, stimulus size, and
stimulus duration.

The field defects characteristic of certain diseases
will be discussed later. For the moment it should
simply be said that a field defect is any statistically and
clinically significant departure from the smooth
shape of the normal hill of vision. Field defects may be
localized, or there may be a general depression of
the whole field. A generally depressed field must be
evaluated for significance, taking into account media
clarity, pupil size, and refraction. Localized field
defects can be described in terms of both size and
depth, and accurate measurements of such defects are
helpful in making a diagnosis. An area of the visual
field where the patient can perceive some stimulus but
where there is less than normal sensitivity is called

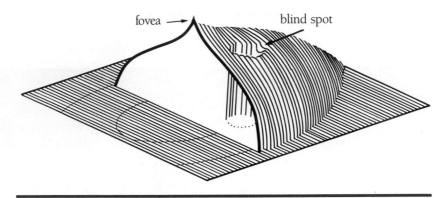

fovea ⟶        blind spot

**Figure 1. The normal hill of vision.** Visual sensitivity is greatest in the fovea where the hill of vision peaks.

a relative scotoma, while an area where the maximum available stimulus is not seen is termed an absolute scotoma. Field defects which are quite evident on perimetric test results may, of course, not be causing the patient any obvious visual problems.

## Static and Kinetic Perimetry

Before the advent of computerized, automated perimetry, manual static perimetry was considered to be a highly sensitive and exact technique, but it was very time-consuming. As a result, it was used mainly in research settings. In recent years, microprocessors have made static perimetry practical in the clinic. It is now possible to present stimuli and record patient responses easily, to improve patient fixation by presenting the stimuli in random order, and to control stimulus duration and timing strictly. Computerization has also improved and expanded the perimetrist's data analysis and storage capabilities.

Most practitioners are experienced in the art and science of manual kinetic perimetry, but they may not have had much experience with static perimetry. The differences between the results of static and kinetic tests reside largely in the increased sophistication of the testing methods the modern static testing instruments use and in their ability to standardize test conditions to a degree that even the most skillful perimetrist would have difficulty matching with manual kinetic instrumentation.

A number of researchers have reported static perimetry to be superior to various methods of kinetic perimetry (figure 2) (Drance et al. 1967; Lynn 1969; Heijl 1976; and Heijl and Lundquist 1983). Katz and Sommer (1986) reported equivalency between automated perimetry and very carefully done kinetic perimetry, although they suggested that automated perimetry is probably superior to routine manual screening methods. On balance, it can be said that automated static perimetry is at least as good as very skillfully performed manual kinetic perimetry, and it is superior to manual perimetry performed under the usually less than ideal conditions of day-to-day clinical practice.

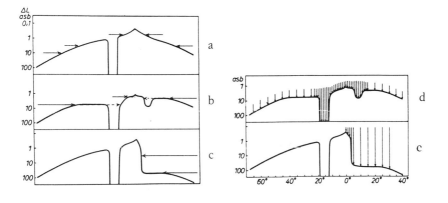

**Figure 2. Static and kinetic perimetry compared.** Slopes and scotomas are shown better by static than kinetic perimetry. Although the normal visual field with its gradual slope and absence of abnormal scotomas is well outlined by kinetic testing (a), the presence of field defects makes this method less precise than static testing. In (b), the flat temporal slope might yield a response at any point between 40° and 12° if the test object were optimum for testing that zone. Nasally, the best chosen kinetic test might be reported anywhere between 25° and 7°, and it would miss the relative scotoma between 7° and 12°. When the slope is steep, kinetic perimetry usually outlines the defect well with a few well- chosen test objects, but the choice is often arbitrary and may, as in (c), fail to reveal the actual steepness of the slope. Static tests elucidate well the flat slopes and small scotomas in (d) and both kinds of slope in (e).
(Figure and caption from Aulhorn and Harms 1967, with permission from S. Karger)

# THE MODERN
# STATIC PERIMETER

**M**ODERN COMPUTERIZED perimeters have evolved
rapidly into sophisticated threshold testing
instruments capable of checking a virtually unlimited
number of point locations with a range of stimulus
sizes and intensities. The Humphrey Field Analyzer, for
example, is a single unit, fully automatic, computerized, projection perimeter. It offers a wide variety
of static field tests, including both threshold measuring
and screening strategies. Test results can be printed
out in several different modes and stored on floppy
disks. The instrument uses standard Goldmann
stimuli and background illumination. It is also
equipped with a set of color filters that can be used for
color perimetry. (See the Humphrey Field Analyzer
*Operator's Manual* for a more complete description of
the instrument and its features.)

## Background Illumination

The Humphrey Field Analyzer uses the 31.5 apostilb
(asb) background illumination that was also used by
the Goldmann perimeter and set as a standard by
the International Perimetric Society (Perimetric Standards 1979). In addition to its familiarity, an advantage
of this background level is that a patient coming in
from a bright room or ordinary outdoor light needs
less time to adapt to the background illumination
before the test can begin. The brighter background also
makes the test less sensitive to stray light in the
room. Perimetry should never be performed in a
brightly lighted room, but with the higher background
it is possible to maintain a low level of ambient light
that allows the office staff to move more freely during
perimetric examinations.

## Stimulus Size and Intensity

The Field Analyzer uses projected stimuli which can
be varied in intensity over a range of more than 5.1

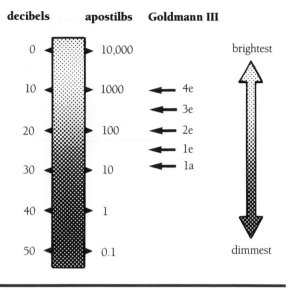

**Figure 3. Stimulus intensity scales compared**

log units (51 decibels) between 0.08 and 10,000
asb. In decibel (dB) notation, the value refers to retinal
sensitivity rather than to stimulus intensity. Therefore,
0 dB corresponds to 10,000 asb, and 51 dB to 0.08
asb (figure 3). The reader more familiar with the
Goldmann system of notation will be relieved to find
that Goldmann filter steps a through e are just
one dB step each. Filters 1 through 4 are five dB steps.
Going from II2e to II3e, then, is a five dB increase
in brightness. Going from I2a to I2c is a two dB
increase.

It is typical in traditional kinetic perimetry to vary
both stimulus size and intensity. In general, computerized static perimetry varies stimulus intensity only,
not stimulus size, during a single test. The Field
Analyzer can cover the whole range of stimulus values,
up to and including the approximate equivalent of
the Goldmann maximum, V4e, without departing from
its standard size III spot. The obvious advantage is
that all results may be compared directly in terms of
brightness; there is no need to convert results from one
spot size to another.

The Field Analyzer offers five sizes of stimuli,
corresponding to the Goldmann perimeter stimuli I

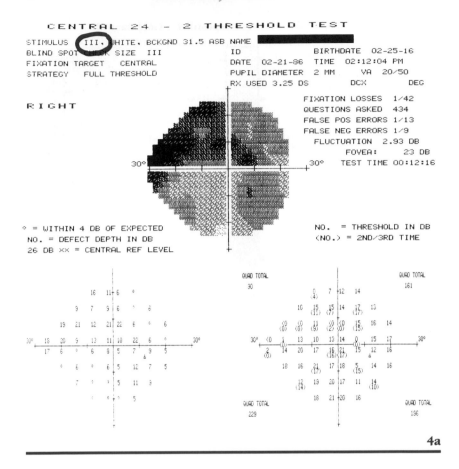

**4a**

through V. This allows maximum flexibility in testing patients with severely disturbed fields and in clinical research. When the equivalent of the Goldmann's maximum stimulus is not sufficient, the Field Analyzer spot size may be switched from size III to size IV or V to provide up to one log unit of stimulus range brighter than that available from the Goldmann perimeter (figure 4). It is also possible to choose a size I or II stimulus if the practitioner so desires. Unless otherwise instructed, the Analyzer will use size III, which is recommended for use with most patients. Since it subtends only 0.43°, the size III is small enough to find even very small scotomata (Flammer et al. 1981), and yet it is large enough to be relatively unaffected by residual refractive error (Sloan 1961; Benedetto and Cyrlin 1985).

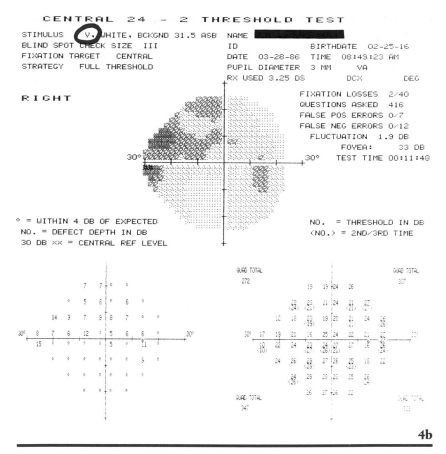

**4b**

**Figure 4.** This 70-year-old patient suffers from both cataract and glaucoma. The patient's right eye was tested first with a size III spot (figure 4a), and then with a size V spot (figure 4b). Note that the use of the size V spot enabled the practitioner to quantify the glaucomatous field defects, while the overall field depression caused by the cataract was more dominant in the test results when the size III spot was used.

Defects that were recorded as absolute when the size III stimulus was used were found to be relative defects when testing was done with the size V stimulus. Testing with the larger spot size makes it possible to follow highly damaged areas and note any progression.

## Stimulus Duration and Randomization

Because fixation is of major importance in eliciting reliable responses from the patient, factors which affect fixation are of key interest in designing a perimeter. Two of those factors are the length of time the stimulus is visible and the order in which stimuli are shown.

Two issues govern the choice of stimulus duration: human reaction time and the principle of temporal summation. The principle of temporal summation holds that for very short durations, the visibility of a stimulus is highly dependent on its exact duration; when a stimulus lasts more than about 0.5 seconds, on the other hand, its visibility is basically independent of duration. That is, it is just as easy to see a spot which is shown for one second as it is to see one which is shown for three seconds (Lynn 1969; Aulhorn and Harms 1972).

Designers of perimeters generally prefer to use as long a stimulus duration as possible in order to minimize the effects of the minor variations in shutter speed which occur in any instrument. However, the stimulus duration must be shorter than the latency time for voluntary eye movements (about 0.25 seconds) so the patient doesn't have time to see the stimulus in the peripheral visual field and look toward it (Perimetric Standards 1979). That would destabilize fixation and confuse the test because the patient's responses would be based on both peripheral and central vision. The Humphrey Field Analyzer uses a stimulus duration of 0.2 seconds.

Fixation also remains more stable if the patient cannot anticipate where the next stimulus is coming from (Heijl and Krakau 1975; Heijl and Drance 1980; Keltner and Johnson 1981). With manual static perimetry, practical reasons of bookkeeping made it impossible to present stimuli in random locations. Automation has removed this barrier to random stimulus presentation, improving fixation and therefore the reliability of the test.

A second advantage of random stimulus presentation is that the testing process cannot affect the local adaptation of the retina. With some patients, showing a strong stimulus in one position and then attempting to determine threshold in the same spot can result in a less accurate finding because the earlier stimuli have bleached away some of the retinal pigment (Aulhorn and Harms 1972; Heijl and Drance 1980). Unlike manual perimetry, automatic computerized perimetry does not test one point or in one area repeatedly in a short period of time.

## Fixation Monitoring

For perimetric results to be valid, the patient must fixate on the fixation target. The ideal fixation device would move the stimuli with the movement of the eye, but at present this type of device is too costly to be practical. Another solution is to monitor the position of the eye continuously and ignore the patient's responses when the eye moves, either from normal head motion such as swallowing or shifting slightly in the chin cup, or from true fixation loss. While currently available methods of continuous eye position monitoring are effective in disallowing false positive responses to stimuli shown when the patient is blinking, they can give false fixation alarms in reaction to small head movements when fixation has, in fact, remained stable. Recent research has also suggested that they are insensitive to movements of 5° or less (Newman 1987).

The designers of the Humphrey Field Analyzer chose the Heijl-Krakau blind spot monitoring technique. This technique provides an index of the quality of patient fixation during an examination by periodically exposing stimuli in the blind spot. Positive responses indicate poor fixation. Because the normal blind spot is approximately 5° by 7°, fixation shifts of only a few degrees can be detected. The blind spot monitoring technique allows the Field Analyzer to make an accurate assessment of patient fixation without the disadvantages of numerous false fixation alarms which tire the patient and can prolong the test.

# 2.

# The Humphrey Field Analyzer Screening and Threshold Strategies

**A**LTHOUGH PROJECTION perimeters such as the Humphrey Field Analyzer can test an almost unlimited number of points in any pattern, factors such as available clinic time and patient fatigue necessarily limit the extent of testing. Therefore, a well-designed instrument must allow the practitioner to concentrate on the area of greatest interest in the testing time available. Computer control and the flexibility of projection perimetry allow the Field Analyzer to tailor the length and point pattern of a test to meet almost any clinical need.

Field Analyzer tests are divided into three categories: threshold measuring programs, screening programs, and the automatic diagnostic program. The latter, an exclusive Humphrey feature, is a sophisticated, space-adaptive strategy which automatically quantifies the depth and breadth of defects detected by a screening test.

# THRESHOLD TESTING

**T**HE HUMPHREY Field Analyzer offers twelve threshold point patterns which can be run with any of three threshold test strategies (see table 1 and figures 5 through 16). The 30-1 and 30-2 central threshold test point patterns are interlocking, as are the 24-1 and 24-2 central test patterns. Separately, each pattern tests points every 6°, but when test results are combined, the effective grid density is 4.2°. Similarly, the 30/60-1 and 30/60-2 peripheral test patterns each have a grid resolution of 12°, and may be merged to give 8.4° resolution. Threshold test results can be printed out in the grayscale format to make interpretation easier (figure 17).

## Table 1. The Humphrey Field Analyzer Threshold Tests

| Test Point Patterns | Print Formats | | | | Test Strategies | | |
|---|---|---|---|---|---|---|---|
| | Numeric | Defect Depth | Gray-scale | Profile | Full Threshold | Full threshold From Prior Data | Fast Threshold |
| Central Tests | | | | | | | |
| Central 24-1 | ✳ | ✳ | ✳ | ✳ | ✳ | ✳ | ✳ |
| Central 24-2 | ✳ | ✳ | ✳ | ✳ | ✳ | ✳ | ✳ |
| Central 30-1 | ✳ | ✳ | ✳ | ✳ | ✳ | ✳ | ✳ |
| Central 30-2 | ✳ | ✳ | ✳ | ✳ | ✳ | ✳ | ✳ |
| Peripheral Tests | | | | | | | |
| Peripheral 30/60-1 | ✳ | ✳ | ✳ | | ✳ | ✳ | ✳ |
| Peripheral 30/60-2 | ✳ | ✳ | ✳ | | ✳ | ✳ | ✳ |
| Nasal Step | ✳ | ✳ | | | ✳ | ✳ | ✳ |
| Temporal Crescent | ✳ | ✳ | | | ✳ | ✳ | ✳ |
| Specialty Tests | | | | | | | |
| Neurological 20 | ✳ | ✳ | | | ✳ | ✳ | ✳ |
| Neurological 50 | ✳ | ✳ | | | ✳ | ✳ | ✳ |
| Central 10-2 | ✳ | ✳ | ✳ | | ✳ | ✳ | ✳ |
| Macula | ✳ | ✳ | | | ✳ | ✳ | ✳ |
| Custom Tests | ✳ | ✳ | | | ✳ | | |

Points can be added to any test pattern or used alone in an arc or profile, as individual points, point clusters, or grids. Single points, grids or point clusters can also be positioned by x,y coordinate.

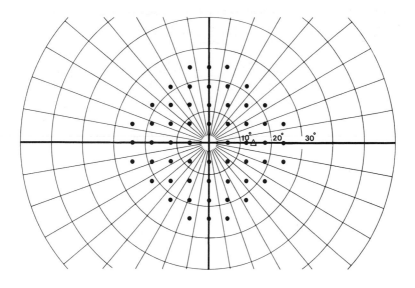

**Figure 5.** Central 24-1 threshold test pattern, right eye

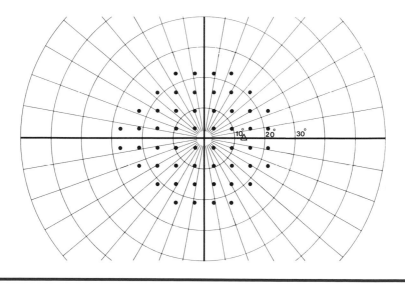

**Figure 6.** Central 24-2 threshold test pattern, right eye

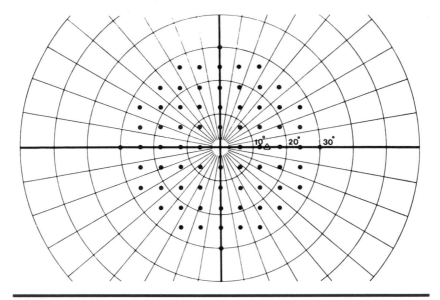

**Figure 7.**  Central 30-1 threshold test pattern, right eye

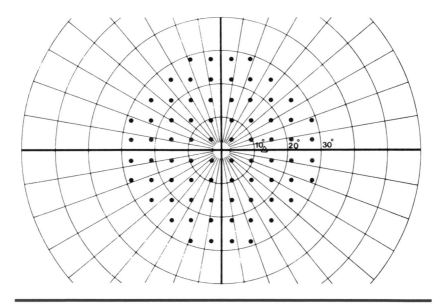

**Figure 8.**  Central 30-2 threshold test pattern, right eye

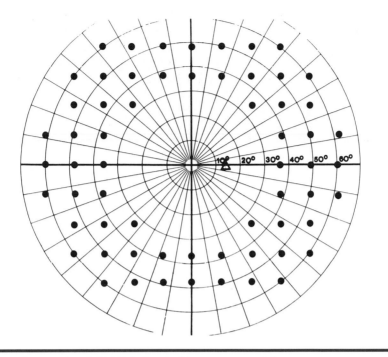

**Figure 9.** Peripheral 30/60-1 threshold test pattern, right eye

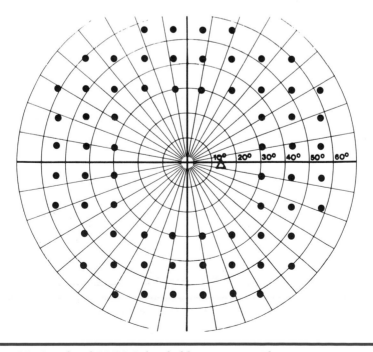

**Figure 10.** Peripheral 30/60-2 threshold test pattern. This same test pattern is used for the peripheral 68 screening test.

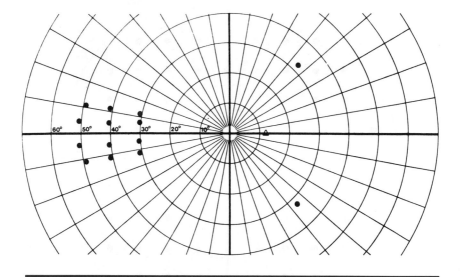

**Figure 11.** Nasal step threshold test pattern, right eye

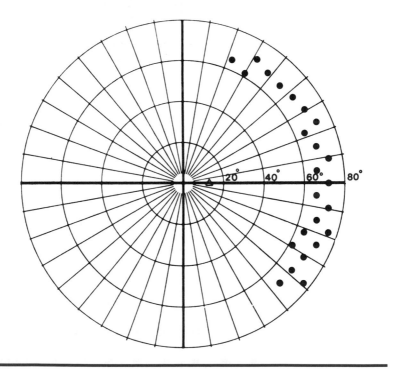

**Figure 12.** Temporal crescent threshold test pattern, right eye

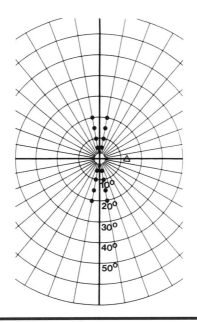

**Figure 13.** Neurological 20 threshold test pattern, right eye

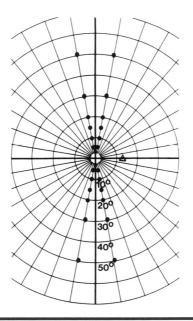

**Figure 14.** Neurological 50 threshold test pattern, right eye

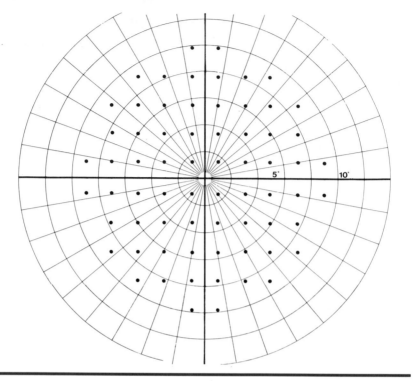

**Figure 15.** Central 10-2 threshold test pattern

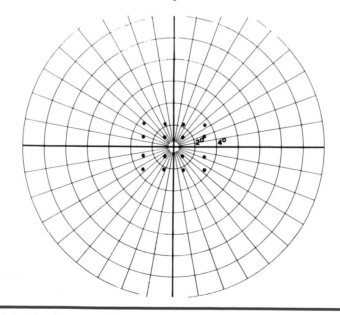

**Figure 16.** Macula threshold test pattern

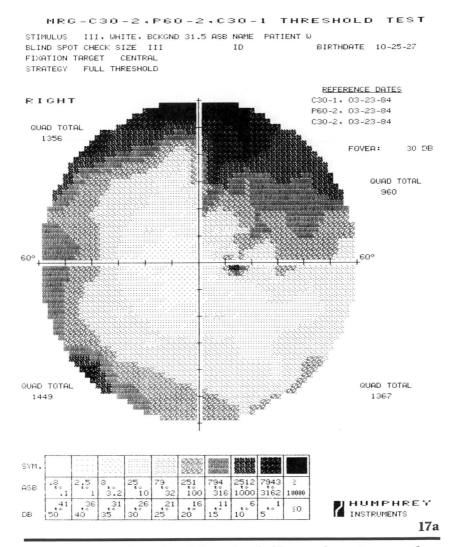

**Figure 17. Merged results of three threshold tests shown in grayscale format.** Merged data are from central 30-1, central 30-2, and peripheral 30/60-2 threshold tests. The fields show bitemporal hemianopia due to pituitary adenoma.

MRG-P60-2,C30-2,C30-1 THRESHOLD TEST

STIMULUS   III, WHITE, BCKGND 31.5 ASB NAME   PATIENT W
BLIND SPOT CHECK SIZE  III              ID              BIRTHDATE  10-25-27
FIXATION TARGET   CENTRAL
STRATEGY   FULL THRESHOLD

REFERENCE DATES
C30-1, 03-23-84
C30-2, 03-23-84
P60-2, 03-23-84

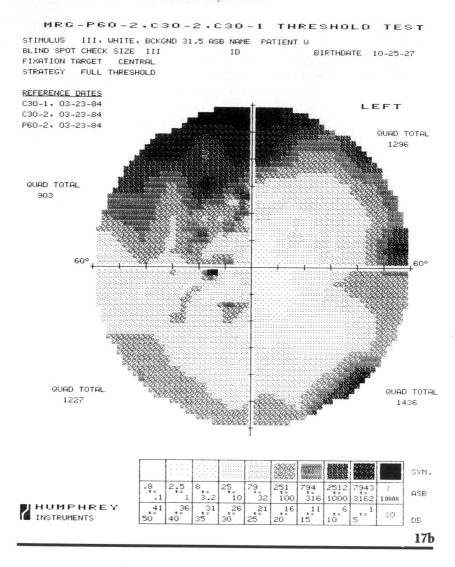

LEFT

QUAD TOTAL
1296

QUAD TOTAL
903

60°                                                           60°

QUAD TOTAL
1227

QUAD TOTAL
1436

| | | | | | | | | | | SYM. |
|---|---|---|---|---|---|---|---|---|---|---|
| .8 to .1 | 2.5 to 1 | 8 to 3.2 | 25 to 10 | 79 to 32 | 251 to 100 | 794 to 316 | 2512 to 1000 | 7943 to 3162 | ≥ 10000 | ASB |
| 41 to 50 | 36 to 40 | 31 to 35 | 26 to 30 | 21 to 25 | 16 to 20 | 11 to 15 | 6 to 10 | 1 to 5 | ≤0 | DB |

**HUMPHREY**
INSTRUMENTS

**17b**

# Determining Threshold

The visual threshold is often thought of as the minimum brightness which the patient can see at a given location in the visual field. The sensitivity of the eye varies from moment to moment and from day to day, as do the alertness of the patient and the criteria the patient uses in answering. Careful design of the instrument and of test method can minimize these effects, but they are always present.

The Humphrey Field Analyzer measures the threshold at a given point by a bracketing, or stairstep, process. It presents the initial stimulus at an intensity slightly brighter than the patient's expected threshold. If the patient sees the spot, the Analyzer decreases the intensity of the stimulus in 4 dB steps in subsequent presentations until the patient does not see it. Then the intensity is increased again in 2 dB steps until the patient sees the stimulus. If, on the other hand, the patient did not see the first stimulus, the same process is performed in reverse. In any case, the last seen value is identified as the patient's threshold at that point.

The Field Analyzer is unique in that whenever the measured threshold departs by 5 dB or more from the expected value for a point in the visual field, the Analyzer rebrackets it. (The expected value is calculated from answers at adjoining points.) Patients naturally make mistakes, and this procedure mimics the strategy used by most human perimetrists who, when presented with an abnormal response from the patient, automatically go back and check to make sure it wasn't a mistake. The second measurement is printed in the test results in parentheses below the first answer; in general, it should be regarded as slightly more valid than the first.

## Threshold Strategies

The first of the three Humphrey Field Analzyer threshold strategies is called full threshold (figure 18). It uses the threshold levels determined at four primary points during test initialization as starting test levels for neighboring points. The results at these neighboring, or secondary, points are then used as starting levels for more neighboring points, and so on. This process makes it possible to threshold a large number of points in the field in a relatively short time.

Two follow-up thresholding strategies, full threshold from prior data and fast threshold, use the Field Analyzer's disk storage capacity to build on information from previous tests of the same patient. The full threshold from prior data strategy begins testing at a level 2 dB brighter than the threshold established by the previous results (figure 19). This saves time in the same way that having a good retinoscopy saves time in subjective refraction.

The fast threshold strategy also begins with stored values from the patient's earlier tests, but instead of retesting to establish a threshold, this strategy tests the field at 2 dB brighter than the stored values. Only the missed points, those which have lost sensitivity since the last test, are thresholded (figure 20). This technique, which is intended for patients who cannot tolerate long threshold testing, is actually a near-threshold supraliminal screening test tailored to the individual patient. It makes it possible to detect disease progression without thresholding points that have not changed.

In addition to the testing strategies, a fluctuation option can be used with any threshold test. When the fluctuation option is chosen, ten pre-selected points are measured twice. The Field Analyzer then makes a calculation based on the consistency of the answers at each point to provide a measure of the reliability of the patient's responses. A small relative defect found in the field of a patient whose fluctuation value shows good consistency is more likely to be real and clinically significant than it would be with a patient whose test results showed poor consistency.

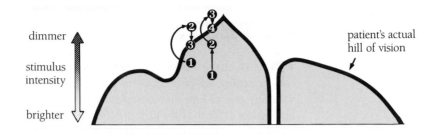

**Figure 18. Full threshold strategy.** This strategy determines retinal sensitivity at each tested point by altering the stimulus intensity in 4 dB steps until the threshold is crossed. It then recrosses the threshold, moving in 2 dB steps, in order to check and refine the accuracy of the measurement.

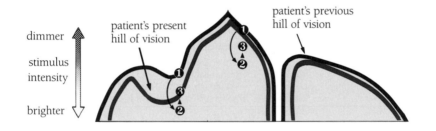

**Figure 19. Full threshold from prior data strategy.** This strategy speeds follow-up testing by using the patient's previous test results as starting points for the new test. Requires Field Analyzer model with optional disk drive data storage system.

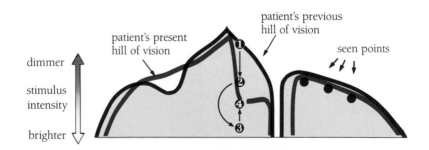

**Figure 20. Fast threshold strategy.** This strategy tests the entire field at 2 dB brighter than stored values from the patient's previous test or tests, and thresholds missed points only. Requires Field Analyzer model with optional disk drive data storage system.

# SCREENING TESTS

**T**HE HUMPHREY Field Analyzer offers eleven screening test point patterns which can be run with any one of four test strategies (see table 2 and figures 10 and 21 through 30). Nine of the patterns examine points where defects are most likely to be found, such as either side of the major meridia and in the arcuate area. The tenth pattern, the 76-point central screening test, is a grid identical to that of the 30-2 central threshold test. This test allows the practitioner who so desires to follow up screening tests with threshold testing at the same points.

**Table 2. The Humphrey Field Analyzer Screening Tests**

| Test Point Patterns | Test Strategies and Recording of Results | | | |
|---|---|---|---|---|
| | Threshold Related (seen or not seen) | Three Zone (seen, relative defect, or absolute defect) | Quantify Defects (depth of defect shown in decibels) | Single Intensity (seen or not seen) |
| Glaucoma Tests | | | | |
|   Armaly Central | ✳ | ✳ | ✳ | ✳ |
|   Armaly Full Field | ✳ | ✳ | ✳ | ✳ |
|   Nasal Step | ✳ | ✳ | ✳ | ✳ |
| Central 30° Tests | | | | |
|   Central 40 | ✳ | ✳ | ✳ | ✳ |
|   Central 76 | ✳ | ✳ | ✳ | ✳ |
|   Central 80 | ✳ | ✳ | ✳ | ✳ |
|   Central 166 | ✳ | ✳ | ✳ | ✳ |
| Peripheral Tests | | | | |
|   Full Field 81 | ✳ | ✳ | ✳ | ✳ |
|   Full Field 120 | ✳ | ✳ | ✳ | ✳ |
|   Full Field 246 | ✳ | ✳ | ✳ | ✳ |
|   Peripheral 68 | ✳ | ✳ | ✳ | ✳ |
| Custom Tests | ✳ | ✳ | ✳ | ✳ |
| Points can be added to any test pattern or used alone in an arc or profile, as individual points, point clusters, or grids. Single points, grids, or point clusters can also be positioned by x,y coordinate. | | | | |
| Automatic Diagnostic | | | ✳ | |

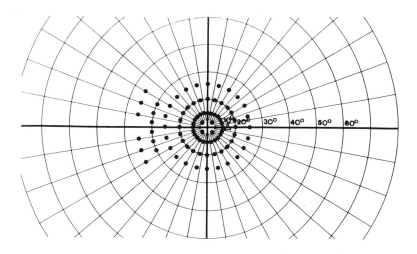

**Figure 21.** Armaly central screening test pattern, right eye

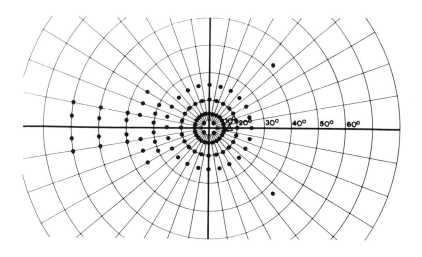

**Figure 22.** Armaly full field screening test pattern, right eye

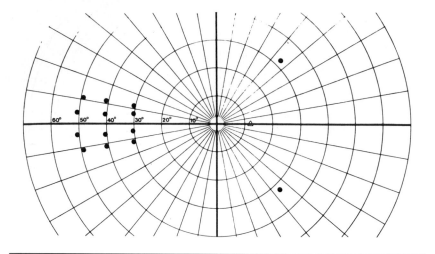

**Figure 23.** Nasal step screening test pattern, right eye

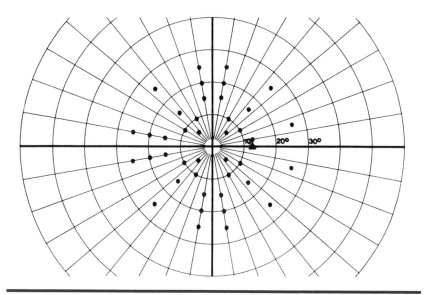

**Figure 24.** Central 40-point screening test pattern, right eye

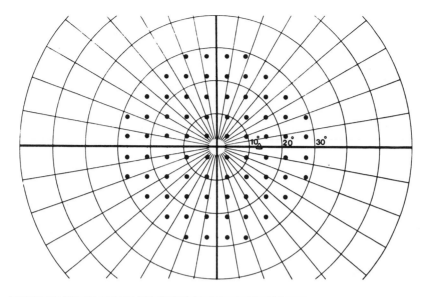

**Figure 25.** Central 76-point screening test pattern, right eye

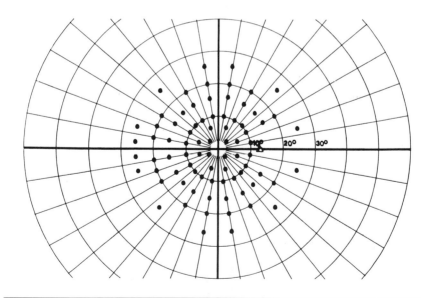

**Figure 26.** Central 80-point screening test pattern, right eye

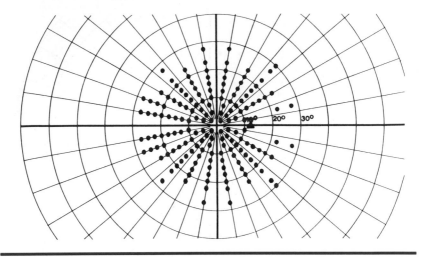

**Figure 27.** Central 166-point screening test pattern, right eye

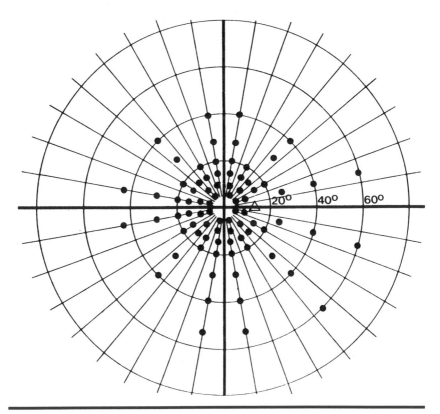

**Figure 28.** Full field 81-point screening test pattern, right eye

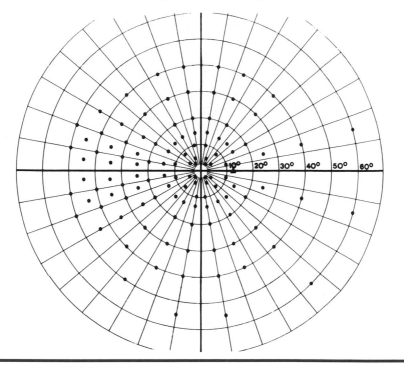

**Figure 29.** Full field 120-point screening test pattern, right eye

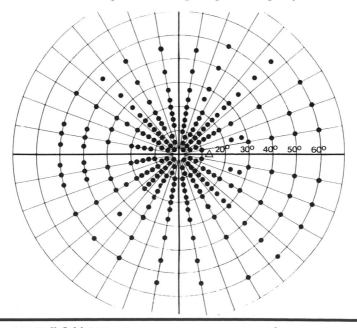

**Figure 30.** Full field 246-point screening test pattern, right eye

# Determining Screening Level

Since screening tests do not determine thresholds at each point, one of the first determinations that must be made concerns the brightness level at which to screen. Obviously, a test which shows stimuli at too bright a level will miss too many relative defects. On the other hand, screening at a very dim level will result in poor test specificity, that is, in too many false positive responses. The Humphrey Field Analyzer screens each point at a brightness level which is 6 dB (0.6 log units) brighter than the expected threshold at that particular point. This value was chosen to provide the best balance between test sensitivity and avoiding false alarms. Stimuli are shown brighter in the periphery and dimmer in the center to accommodate the natural slope in the hill of vision.

It may be helpful here to explain how the Field Analyzer determines the standard for what is normal for a given patient, that is, the point-by-point baseline to which the 6 dB correction may be applied. The designers of some automatic perimeters have measured a large number of normal subjects and used the point-by-point average of their answers, usually adjusted for age, as the baseline.

The Field Analyzer goes one step further. Every test begins with an initialization procedure that determines a threshold level for one point in each quadrant of the central field. Then because there is wide disparity among normal patier.ts and averages can be misleading, the Field Analyzer adjusts the normal baseline up or down based on the answers at the first four points tested (figure 31). This forms the reference hill of vision, automatically corrected for the patient's age, pupil size, media clarity, and general responsiveness. The instrument also prints out the height of the patient's hill of vision, called the central reference level, so that the doctor knows the brightness level at which the test was run. It is possible to set the central reference level manually if the practitioner so desires.

In order to catch the patient with a strongly depressed field, a limit is put on the amount which the baseline may be shifted. If the patient's central reference level is below 26 dB, the value appears in the test results as 26 dB XX to let the doctor know that the actual value is below that level, and the screening test is run at a brightness appropriate for a central reference level of 26 dB. A central reference level of less than 26 dB is likely to mean a significantly depressed or constricted field.

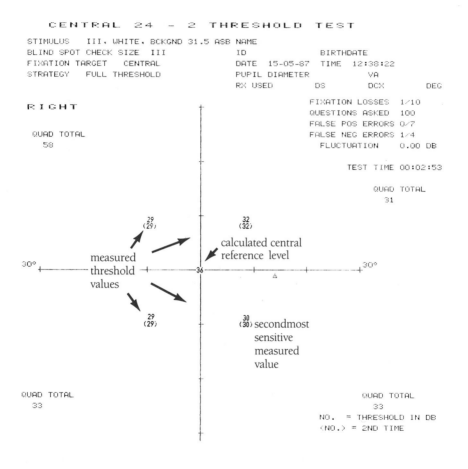

**Figure 31. Calculating the predicted hill of vision.** Four primary points, one in each quadrant, are thresholded. The secondmost sensitive value is used to calculate the expected height of the hill of vision, known as the central reference level. Screening test stimuli are then presented 6 dB brighter than the patient's calculated hill of vision.

## Screening Strategies

The Humphrey Field Analyzer offers three main screening strategies which can be used with any of the standard screening test point patterns. The first is called the threshold-related strategy (figure 32). With this strategy, if the patient sees a point the first or second time it is tested, the area is recorded as normal. When the patient doesn't see the stimulus, the point is tested again to make sure the miss wasn't a mistake. If the point is missed a second time, the Field Analyzer registers a miss and moves on. Since screening with this strategy is done at an intensity 6 dB brighter than the expected threshold, missed points are known to be at least 6 dB deep.

Two other Humphrey screening strategies give additional information about missed points. The three-zone strategy records points as seen, relative defect, and absolute defect (figure 33). It retests any missed points at 10,000 asb. If the point is seen at that level, it is recorded as a relative defect; if it is not seen, it is recorded as an absolute defect.

The quantify defects strategy provides additional information (figure 34). Like the three-zone strategy, it gains this extra information at the expense of extra testing time on patients with abnormal fields. However, normal patients take no more time, and many practitioners feel that the extra time is more than justified for those patients who miss points. When the quantify defects strategy is used, all missed points are thresholded and the depth of the defect is recorded on the test results in decibels.

One other screening strategy is available for specialized applications. When the practitioner would like to check the whole field at one intensity, the single-intensity strategy can be used.

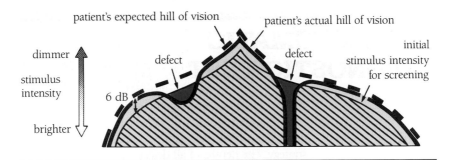

**Figure 32. Threshold-related screening strategy.** This strategy records tested points as seen or not seen. Screening is done at an intensity 6 dB brighter than the expected threshold, and points missed twice at that level are recorded as defects.

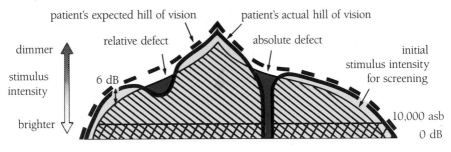

**Figure 33. Three-zone screening strategy.** This strategy records tested points three ways: seen, relative defect, or absolute defect. Screening is done at an intensity 6 dB brighter than the expected threshold, and points missed twice are retested at 10,000 asb. A point seen on retesting is recorded as a relative defect; if it is not seen, it is recorded as an absolute defect.

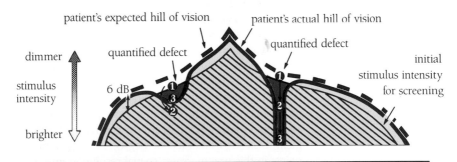

**Figure 34. Quantify defects screening strategy.** This strategy provides additional information. Screening is done at 6 dB brighter than the expected threshold. Points missed twice at the screening level are thresholded. For all missed points the depth of the defect, relative to the expected threshold, is recorded in dB.

# THE AUTOMATIC DIAGNOSTIC TEST

**T**HE FIELD Analyzer's automatic diagnostic test is a screening procedure that provides even more information than the quantify defects screening strategy. The depths of all defects are quantified, as they are with the quantify defects strategy, and up to ten additional points are added to the pattern around each missed point. The additional points are screened and recorded as seen or missed. This gives the practitioner a quick idea of both the depth and size of the defect. If more than forty defects are found in the field, a warning message appears on the screen, and the depths of the defects are not quantified. It is assumed in such cases that quantifying more than forty points would fatigue the patient and that the practitioner would prefer to spend the time running a test with the full threshold strategy.

# CUSTOM TESTS

**T**HE FIELD Analyzer's standard features include a custom test option that can be used for both screening and thresholding. It allows the perimetrist to focus in on an area where a first test indicated defects. The practitioner may add points to any of the Field Analyzer's standard screening or threshold test patterns, or design a custom point pattern that can be used alone (figures 35 and 36). The points can be added both centrally or peripherally in a grid pattern, as single points, in point clusters, or along a meridian or an arc. It is possible, for example, to add points along any profile in the central field, spacing them as close together as one degree. Adding extra points in this way increases spatial resolution in pathological areas, providing a more exact measurement of the true size of a field defect.

Humphrey Field Analyzers with software released in 1986 or later can store any custom point pattern which the practioner has designed and wishes to keep and reuse.

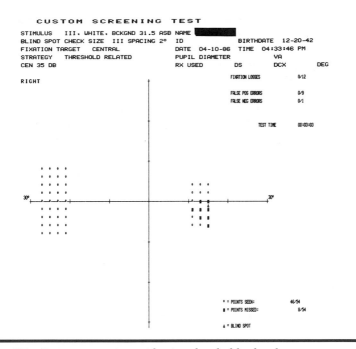

**Figure 35.** Custom screening grid using threshold-related strategy

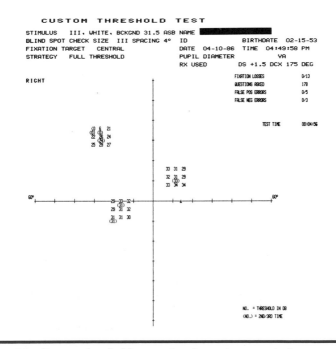

**Figure 36.** Custom threshold test point cluster in numeric format.

# 3.

# Using the Humphrey Field Analyzer in the Clinic

**T**HE FLEXIBILITY and range of the Field Analyzer make it possible to test fields efficiently for almost any purpose. The shorter screening tests are thorough enough to alert the doctor to the presence of field defects without tiring the patient or using too much clinic time. When a problem is detected, any of the full range of tests can be employed in the diagnostic process. Finally, there are highly specialized test patterns and strategies to use in following up pathological fields.

# TEST RELIABILITY: THE PATIENT AND THE PERIMETRIST

**P**ATIENT COOPERATION is the key to test reliability. The perimetrist's instructions and encouragement are important to the patient's attitude and ability to be a good test subject. Patients who have never had any field screening at all should receive careful instruction before they take a test with the Field Analyzer. It is

crucial for the new patient to realize that the test is not
a game in which the the objective is to look around
the bowl in order to see all the lights. We recommend
that the perimetrist read the standard instructions
on the Patient Instruction Screen to the patient.
To avoid compromising the consistency of test results,
the perimetrist should develop a consistent method
of reading the instructions so that the patient is
instructed in the same manner for each test.

Patients who have experience with screening tests
and with Goldmann kinetic perimetry need to
understand that a static threshold test is a different
kind of test. These patients are used to the success of
finally seeing the spot at each stimulus presentation
and sometimes become anxious when they don't have
this satisfaction. During a Field Analyzer threshold
test, more than half the stimuli will not be seen
because the instrument is bracketing to determine
threshold or checking for false positive responses and
fixation losses. Many of the stimuli which are seen
are just barely visible. The perimetrist should make it
clear that the test is pushing the limit of the patient's
vision, and that no one is expected to see the stimulus
every time.

When the Analyzer indicates fixation errors, they
may be caused by poor patient fixation, a "trigger
happy" patient, or a mistake in locating the blind spot.
Sometimes patient errors during the blind spot
plotting process can mislead the Analyzer about the
location of the blind spot, resulting in a poor fixation
score. Replotting the blind spot may help. If fixation
remains poor, the perimetrist can reinstruct the patient
or allow a short rest. Most patients improve their
fixation when they understand the nature and objectives
of the test, and fixation generally improves after
reinstruction.

For patients with macular disease or other central
scotomata, it may be necessary to switch to one
of the two fixation diamonds. In such cases, the patient
looks at the apparent center of a four-point pattern
of light-emitting diodes; central vision is not required.
The peripheral fixation diamonds are used with all
patients for foveal testing.

The perimetrist should always make sure the patient
is seated as comfortably as possible and be sure to

watch for factors such as arthritis that could make it difficult for the patient to press the button. (Full instructions for running demonstration tests to check fixation and administering Humphrey Field Analyzer field tests are found in the *Operator's Manual*.)

There is a widespread subjective impression that after six or seven minutes a patient begins to tire and do more poorly on a visual field test. In fact, patients commonly do perfectly well on tests lasting up to twenty minutes or longer. The visual field itself is remarkably stable in normal subjects over testing periods as long as half an hour (Heijl 1977; Holmin and Krakau 1979). The patient should definitely be informed in advance that it is normal for the background to seem to change or for the fixation point to seem to move. During a long test some patients may even see occasional spots of light that do not come from the instrument, but these entopic phenomena disturb the test results less than one would think. Elderly patients especially sometimes tire during longer tests, and if the patient would like to rest, it is fine to hold the button down and take a break from time to time.

One advantage of automated, computerized perimetry is that once the demonstration test has shown that the patient understands the test properly, the perimetrist does not have to watch the whole test, especially with an experienced patient. Occasionally telling a new patient when fixation is good can provide a helpful feeling of success, and some practitioners do feel the perimetrist should monitor the entire test with all patients. Another point of view, however, holds that a very active perimetrist can compromise the objectivity of the test. If, during the course of the test, the perimetrist tells the patient to look especially hard or reminds the patient to press the button even if the stimulus seems weak, it is possible to change the patient's criteria for what he or she considers a seen point. This can eliminate some of the consistency that is a major advantage of automatic perimetry. Perhaps the main point to emphasize is that careful instruction, demonstration and observation at the beginning of the test will save much time and generally improve the quality of results.

Clearly, a good reason to start new patients on a screening test is that the screening test is easier to take than a threshold test. A screening test takes less time, and the patient will see almost all the stimuli. For new patients, the easier the test, the more reliable the results tend to be. So, while the doctor might in theory find a threshold test more informative, in practice, the results from a first-time threshold test are sometimes questionable. Many practitioners have concluded that it is better to give a screening test, which will detect any sizable field defects, and to order a threshold test later if further information is needed.

# BASIC SCREENING RECOMMENDATIONS

T HE PRACTITIONER who runs visual field screening tests on patients in all age groups should know that the probability of finding disease in a general population is small. The incidence of glaucoma has been shown to be slightly higher in the section of the population over fifty-two years of age, but definite glaucoma will still be found in only a small percentage of patients screened (Liebowitz et al. 1980). The main causes of clinically significant field defects are neurological disease and glaucoma (Hard-Boberg and Wirtschafter 1985). It can probably be safely stated that most other consequential conditions produce distinctive diagnostic signs and symptoms other than visual field defects.

One important clinical question that has not been clearly resolved is how often field defects are missed if only the central 30° of the field is examined. Some reseachers hold that it is very rare for field defects caused by glaucoma to appear in the peripheral field unless the central field is also disturbed (Le Blanc et al. 1985), but others disagree (Caprioli and Spaeth 1985). Field defects of neurological origin tend to be best detected in the central 30° (Frisen 1985; Hard-Boberg and Wirtschafter 1985; Mills 1985). The consensus among researchers is that given a limited amount of testing time, it is best to concentrate on the central field. Once loss in the central field has been established, there is, of course, value in quantifying visual field loss in the periphery.

Unless there is a specific reason to begin with a more extensive test, a 76-point central field test is often the best way to begin with a new patient. The number of tested points is probably sufficient for most applications, and the pattern is identical to the 30-2 threshold test, making it possible to threshold test any missed points later. If defects are found in the central field, then it may be worthwhile to test the peripheral field as well. When the focus of interest is the peripheral field, the peripheral 68 test is a good choice. The pattern is identical to the 30/60-2 threshold test, which can be used if follow-up threshold testing seems appropriate.

For patients who cannot complete a 76-point central test, the central 40-point test is the next choice. Or, for patients who can tolerate a longer test, test sensitivity can be improved slightly with the full field 120-point exam. While sensitivity can be improved a bit more with the 246-point full field screening test, a central 30-2 threshold test takes the same amount of time and provides better information about most conditions.

The Armaly central and Armaly full field patterns are well-established means of detecting glaucomatous defects, offering 90% to 95% detection rates, respectively (Rock, Drance and Morgan 1971; 1973). It has traditionally been held that nasal steps can occur both centrally and peripherally, and it may be of benefit to check for peripheral nasal steps, but as explained previously, the benefits of such testing are not now clearly established. The nasal step threshold test can be added as a quick peripheral check to any of the Field Analyzer's central screening tests to detect the small percentage of glaucomatous defects which do appear in the peripheral field.

# BASIC THRESHOLDING RECOMMENDATIONS

U NLESS A different course of action is already indicated, it is best to begin thresholding glaucoma patients or suspects with the 30-2 threshold test in order to concentrate on the central field and to test sensitivities at points which straddle the horizontal and vertical meridia. When patient fatigue is a significant factor, the 24-2 threshold test provides almost as much information as the 30-2, and it takes less than three-quarters of the time (figure 37). For patients with a clear central visual field but suspicious pressures or disk signs, the nasal step test is a quick way to make sure that the patient does not belong to the small percentage of glaucoma patients who exhibit peripheral field loss only.

Neurological field defects are more predictable in location than those caused by glaucoma. Almost all conduction-type neurological field defects occur in the central field, and as a general rule, differences between right and left fields become more pronounced closer to fixation. The difference across the vertical meridian is most informative, and a great deal can be learned from simply thresholding points on each side of that meridian. When the central field is examined with a very sensitive threshold test such as the Humphrey Field Analyzer 30-2 or 24-2, it is usually unnecessary to test the peripheral field as well (Frisen 1985; Hard-Boberg and Wirtschafter 1985; Mills 1985).

Among the general purpose threshold tests, the 30-2 or 24-2 are well suited to detect defects caused by neurological disease because they include points on either side of the vertical meridian. They also give additional information on the shape and extent of any detected defects. However, patients with neurological diseases are often quite ill and easily fatigued. When a longer test is not possible, one of the abbreviated threshold tests such as the neurological 20 or neurological 50, which test only on either side of the vertical meridian, can provide useful information about hemianopic defects in minimal time. If the neurological tests prove too taxing, the next choice is a short, central field screening test. Almost all neurological defects that traditional manual kinetic perimetry, well-performed, would be likely to detect would probably also be clearly indicated on any of the Analyzer's central screening tests.

The 30-1 threshold test includes points on the horizontal and vertical meridia. The point pattern of the 30-1 interlocks with that of the 30-2 to yield a grid of points spaced every 4.2°. When the two tests are merged, using the Field Analyzer's merge feature, the result is a very high resolution picture of threshold levels in the central 30° of the visual field. This sort of detailed testing can be very helpful in establishing a baseline for following up small field defects. The 24-1 pattern combines with the 24-2 in the same way, again providing 4.2° resolution.

When the practitioner suspects a disease which affects the peripheral visual field, the 30/60-2 is the examination of choice. Like the central threshold tests, the 30/60-1 and 30/60-2 peripheral tests can be merged to provide a detailed examination of the peripheral visual field, giving 8.4° resolution.

Finally, custom points can be used alone in an area where field defects are suspected, or they can be added to threshold tests as single points, point clusters, grids, profiles or arcs. In the past, profile tests along the 45-225° and 135-315° meridia have been used as a standard part of very ambitious glaucoma perimetry, even though they were quite time-consuming to perform manually. The Field Analyzer offers rapid automatic testing along these and any other meridia the practitioner would like to check.

The custom patterns provide an efficient means of evaluating questionable portions of the visual field in detail to determine whether an apparent field loss is consistent without repeating the entire test. Take, for example, a test which shows a field defect which is so small it only covers one of the points. If no more testing is done, the doctor will have data for only

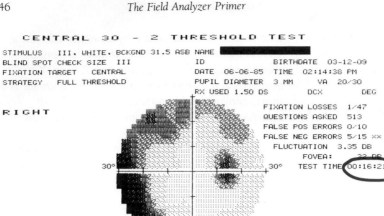

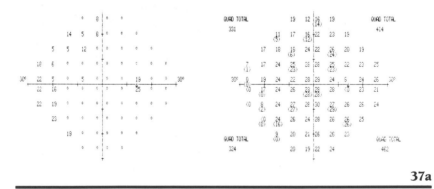

**37a**

one disturbed point and may not be sure how to interpret it. Adding custom test points in a cluster or high-density grid around a small, questionable area is a good way to determine whether the single missed point represents a true field defect and to define the borders of the affected area quickly (see figures 35 and 36).

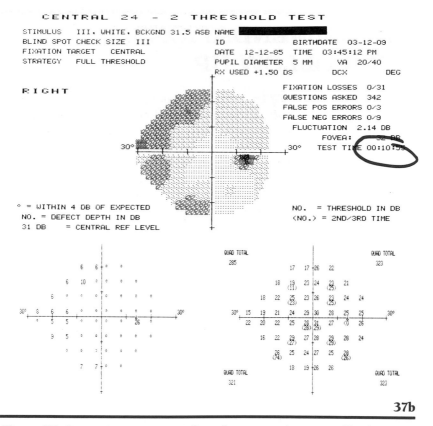

**37b**

**Figure 37.** In certain cases, especially with patients who tire readily, there is an advantage to using the 24-2 threshold test. The practitioner who has been following this easily fatigued 77-year-old glaucoma patient knows that there is a binasal depression as defined by the 30-2 results shown in figure 37a. The practitioner has chosen to follow this particular patient with the 24-2 threshold test pattern (figure 37b) because it takes significantly less test time and still retains the nasal step points in the outer 30° area.

This example also illustrates the variability often seen in pathological visual fields. The nasal step area shows much deeper losses in the first test than in the second.

# RECOMMENDATIONS FOR FOLLOW UP

T HE MOST important recommendation for following
up detected field defects is *do not* change the
test point pattern or stimulus characteristics. It is
important that the data remain comparable from
test to test. Some doctors have asked whether there is
any benefit in retesting with a different test, for
instance, following a 30-2 with a 30-1 to give more
spatial resolution, rather than with another 30-2
to give more threshold information. Because repeata-
bility and comparability of data are such important
factors in retesting, the first priority recommendation
is to use the same test. If there is time for additional
testing, running a 30-1 test and merging the results
with those from the 30-2 can provide valuable
detail. It is also possible to focus down on the area of
concern with a custom test.

   Field defects should be followed with threshold
measuring techniques, if possible. In glaucoma,
for example, field defects become deeper more often
than they enlarge (Mikelberg and Drance 1984),
and that type of change is much easier to appreciate
on a threshold test, although it can also be detected by
a screening test run with the quantify defects
strategy. With elderly, easily fatigued patients who
cannot complete a longer test, it is better to follow up
with screening tests than not follow up at all.

   When a patient has advanced glaucoma and large
field defects with only small but very important
remnants of the central visual field remaining, it is
vital to follow that small area closely. The patient's
condition may require the practitioner to rely on
data from only four or five points. Because there is a
great deal of variability in highly degraded fields, there
is a risk of missing significant deterioration. It might
be an advantage to follow such fields with a high-
density custom grid. The 2° spacing of the macula test
provides the detailed information needed to determine
whether the defect is in danger of impinging on the
fovea. Remember that because glaucoma and some

other diseases cause visual field defects to vary, a series of measurements should be taken over time to allow the practitioner to determine whether the results of a given field test represent variation rather than genuine progression or regression of the disease. (For further discussion of following up glaucomatous defects see page 82.)

## When In Doubt, Retest

It is sometimes hard to know whether very small indications of field defects in the printouts represent testing uncertainty or disease. Retesting is the best way to differentiate between the two. The probability that a discrete area of lowered sensitivity in the visual field represents disease rather than variation increases significantly if test results are reproducible. The defect need not have exactly the same appearance in subsequent tests, but if there is a disturbance in the same area when the test is repeated, it is likely that there is a true field defect.

# USING THE MERGE, AVERAGE, AND COMPARE PROGRAMS

ONE STANDARD feature of the Humphrey Field Analyzer is a package of programs intended to assist the practitioner in interpreting follow-up test results. The Analyzer's merge feature has been described earlier. Briefly, it makes it possible to merge threshold test results from test patterns designed with interlocking points, such as the 30-1 and 30-2, or to combine a central and a peripheral test such as the 30-2 and the 30/60-2.

The average feature establishes a good baseline for a patient by averaging a number of tests which can then be used to judge disease progression in the future. Averaging is recommended for use in cases where it is particularly important to be able to judge the progression of a disease even when it is subtle.

The compare feature allows the practitioner to compare a given test result against a previously established baseline. Running two sets of averaged fields and then comparing them is a sensitive way of determining whether a patient's condition is deteriorating.

The Field Analyzer's Statpac program, which is discussed in detail in chapter 6, is another useful tool in follow-up testing. Statpac can be used to perform a statistical analysis of a series of tests, yielding a sensitive and highly informative picture of changes in the patient's visual field over time.

# 4.

# Reading the Field Analyzer Printouts

**T** FIRST thing to do in learning to interpret data from a computerized perimeter is to become familiar with the ways in which test results can be printed. Humphrey Field Analyzer test results can be printed out in five threshold test formats, three screening test formats, or three Statpac formats. The threshold and screening test result formats are discussed in this chapter, and Statpac printouts are discussed in chapter 6.

# THRESHOLD TEST PRINTOUTS

**H** UMPHREY FIELD ANALYZER threshold test results can be printed on a grayscale, which gives a picture resembling isopters; a defect depth grid with the depths of defects indicated in decibels; and a numeric grid with threshold levels shown in decibels. The three-in-one printout, which includes all three methods of presentation on a single sheet of paper, is available for most commonly used Humphrey Field Analyzer threshold tests. It is also possible to print interpolated results along a given meridian in profile form (figure 39).

Figure 38 is an example of a three-in-one printout of the results of a Humphrey Field Analyzer threshold test on Patient A's left eye. The top line tells the type of test used to gather the data, a 30-2 central threshold test. The first five lines on the right give patient information, and the basic parameters used in the test appear on the left. The word LEFT in capital letters indicates which eye was tested.

Three of the next six lines of information that appear on the left side of the page indicate the reliability of this particular test. There were two fixation losses out of 45 fixation checks, and no false positive and one false negative responses out of four and nine checks, respectively. A total of 535 stimuli were shown to the patient, and the fluctuation test was not used. If the fluctuation test had been turned on, a fluctuation value would appear instead of the word "off." The patient took 15 minutes and 49 seconds to complete this particular test. The typical 30-2 threshold test takes about 13 minutes; a patient with a very disturbed field will take longer. The full threshold from prior data and fast threshold strategies reduce the time required for follow-up tests.

The grayscale representation of the patient's visual field provides an immediate idea of the size and seriousness of the field defects present. A comparative scale which relates the grayscale to decibels is shown at the bottom of the page. Each step of the pattern corresponds to a change of 5 dB in sensitivity. The borders between gray tones are roughly analogous to isopters measured every 5 dB. Remember, a 5 dB change in brightness is approximately equivalent to a change of one Goldmann stimulus size.

The defect depth grid shown in the lower left section of the page indicates normal points with ○. Points which may be significantly abnormal are indicated by positive numbers which represent the defect depth in decibels. The height of this particular patient's hill of vision, determined during the test initialization process, is given as the central reference level. The blind spot location on this and several other types of Field Analyzer printouts is indicated by Δ.

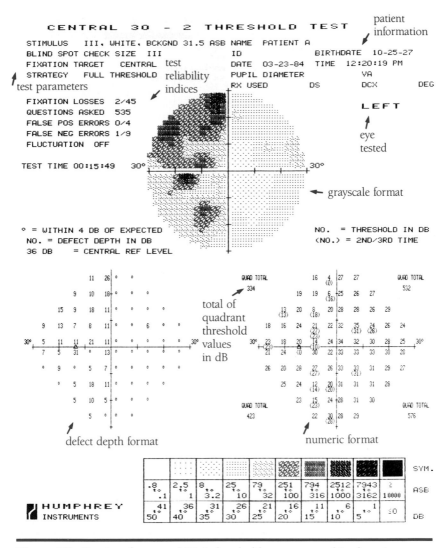

**Figure 38.** Results of a central 30-2 threshold test presented in three-in-one format, pituitary adenoma patient

The numeric grid shown in the lower right section of the page gives the threshold in decibels for all points checked. Points which are at least 5 dB less sensitive than expected are checked a second time, and the value shown in parentheses represents the threshold found on the second check. This double-

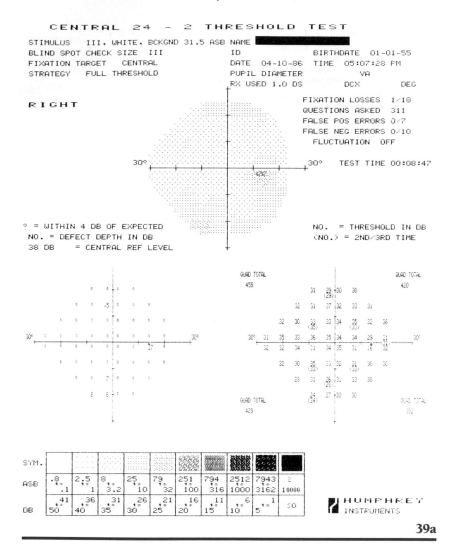

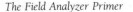

checking verifies unexpected answers and helps the practitioner differentiate between patient errors and true field defects. In general, the second values can be considered slightly more accurate than the first value.

The numbers which appear just outside each quadrant of the numeric grid are quad totals, or summations of the threshold values determined in each quadrant. These numbers, which will not be the same for each quadrant, can be useful in comparing several tests on the same patient taken over time.

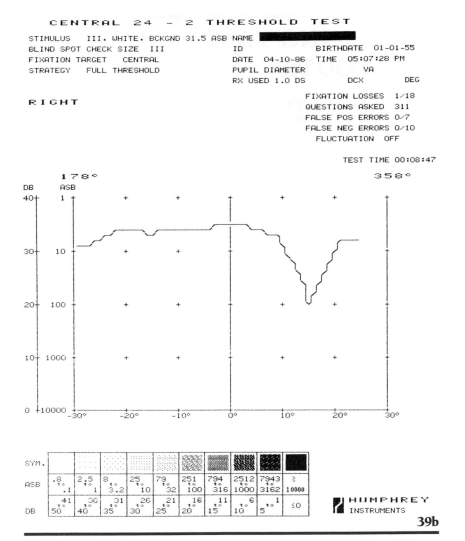

**Figure 39.** These central 24-2 results are slightly suspicious because of the three points with somewhat decreased sensitivities infero-nasally (figure 39a). Further testing is probably called for. It is not unusual, however, to see such results in normal patients. Results along the 178°-358° meridian from the same test are shown in profile format in figure 39b.

# SCREENING TEST PRINTOUTS

**T**HE SCREENING test printouts use symbols for seen and missed points. When the test is run according to the threshold-related strategy (figure 40), the missed point is indicated by the "not seen" symbol (■). With the three-zone strategy (figure 41), a missed point is identified either by ■, meaning absolute defect in this case; or by X, meaning relative defect. When the quantify defects strategy is used, numbers indicating the depth of the defect in decibels replace the missed point symbol (figure 42).

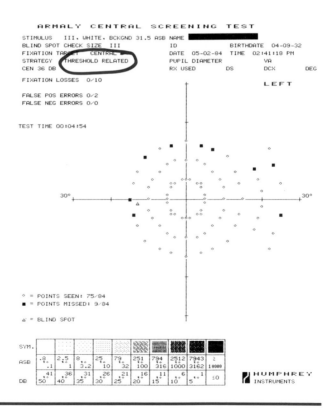

**Figure 40.** Armaly central screening test using threshold-related strategy, glaucoma patient

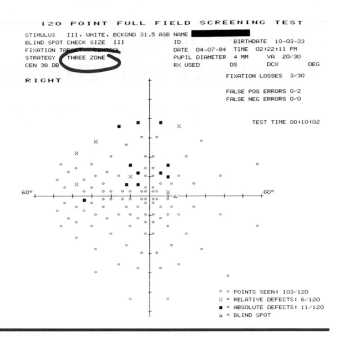

**Figure 41.** Full field 120-point screening test using three-zone strategy, glaucoma patient

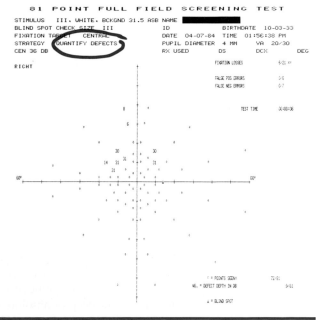

**Figure 42.** Full field 81-point screening test using quantify defects strategy, glaucoma patient

# INDICES OF THE
# RELIABILITY OF THE TEST

I N INTERPRETING test results the first thing to do is
evaluate the factors that indicate the reliability
of this particular patient on this particular test. These
factors are the fixation losses score, the number of
false positive and false negative errors, fluctuation, and
any information about the patient the perimetrist
thought noteworthy. If these indices suggest the data
are unreliable, the test results cannot be of much
help in diagnosis and the patient should be retested.

## Fixation Losses

The fixation losses value is an indication of how
well the patient fixates, and the lower it is, the more
confidence one can have in the test results. During a
test, the Humphrey Field Analyzer periodically
checks the patient's fixation by presenting stimuli in
the blind spot. If the patient responds, the Analyzer
records a fixation loss. If the fixation losses value is
above 20%, there are reasons for concern, and
XX appears next to the value on the printout to draw
the practitioner's attention.

When fixation is poor, two possibilities should be
considered. The most likely one, of course, is that the
patient is not fixating well. In that case, the test can
miss small field defects, and the depth of large defects
will usually be underestimated because the patient
will occasionally see a stimulus with a more sensitive
part of the retina than would be the case if fixation
were good.

The second reason for a poor fixation score could
be a misplotted blind spot. Check how well the
blind spot has been defined in the numeric threshold
printout. If there is a high fixation losses score and
none of the thresholded points around the physiological
blind spot show deep or absolute defects, that
probably indicates poor fixation. However, a poor
fixation score plus a blind spot that is well-defined by
the thresholded points may mean that the patient

made too many errors during the blind spot mapping process at the beginning of the test, not that fixation is poor. Running the short demonstration test before beginning actual testing should help forestall this problem.

## False Negative and False Positive Errors

Occasionally during each test, the projector moves as if to present a stimulus but does not do so. If the patient responds, a false positive error is recorded. At other times a stimulus which is much brighter than threshold is presented in an area where sensitivity has already been determined. If the patient does not respond, a false negative error is recorded. The total number of both types of errors appears on the printout. A high false positive score indicates that the patient is "trigger happy," and a high false negative score may indicate a fatigued or inattentive patient.

## Fluctuation

When the fluctuation test is turned on during threshold testing, the threshold is measured twice at ten predetermined point locations. The Field Analyzer then calculates a fluctuation value on the basis of the differences between the first and second measurements at each of the ten points. This value is an index of how reliable a patient's responses were during the test. A patient who is very consistent will have a low fluctuation value, while a patient whose responses vary significantly during the test will have a high value. A high fluctuation value may be the first sign of glaucomatous field loss in patients who are otherwise reliable perimetric subjects. It is also associated with established field loss in reliable test subjects. On the other hand, a high fluctuation value may simply indicate that the patient is inattentive or does not understand the test.

When test results are analyzed with Statpac, the fluctuation value is used as one basis for calculating another index of reliability, CPSD. It is therefore important to leave the fluctuation option on during threshold testing. See chapter 6 for more information.

## Perimetrist's Comments

In some cases it may be important for the perimetrist to record some aspects of the patient's behavior during the test. A patient who seems confused or possibly disoriented may be a much less reliable test subject than an alert, attentive patient. A patient who has to pause and rest often may need to be retested another time with a shorter, less comprehensive test. Data from an accurate short test are more useful than unreliable data from a more comprehensive test. The perimetrist should record the presence of any physical condition, such as extreme weakness, head tremors or arthritis, which might have adversely affected the validity of the procedure.

# 5.

# Interpreting Test Results: Hallmarks of Pathological Fields

**M**OST PRACTITIONERS are accustomed to interpreting visual fields represented as isopters. This method of representation, while appropriate for kinetic perimetry, is less suited to the data yielded by static perimetry, which consist of numbers representing thresholds at tested points.

The practitioner who has gained some familiarity with the ways Field Analyzer test results are presented will soon notice that field loss measured on a static perimeter looks much as it does when measured on a kinetic instrument. The language is slightly different, but the principles are the same. This is especially apparent if one compares kinetic isopters with static threshold grayscale printouts. For example, the field loss in the nasal area in figure 43 appears as a darkening of the grayscale printout and as a contraction of the kinetic isopters in the nasal area on the Goldmann field chart. Similarly, the Humphrey Field Analyzer grayscale printout of a hemianopic field will show the left or right half of the field to be considerably darker than the opposite side, instead of the perhaps more familiar picture of kinetic isopters bending sharply at the vertical meridian.

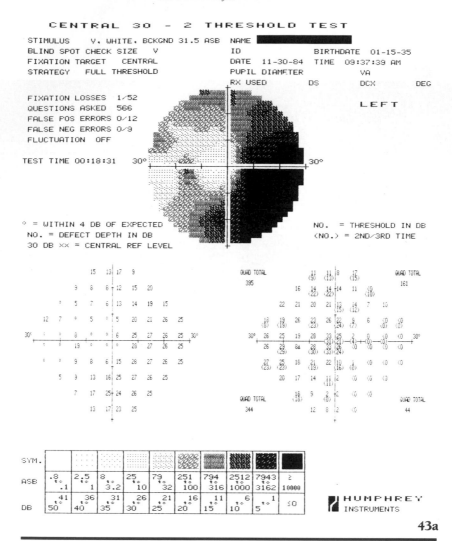

**Figure 43.** The results of a Humphrey Field Analyzer central 30-2 threshold test (figure 43a) can be compared with those of a Goldmann manual kinetic test (figure 43b) run on the left eye of a 50-year-old man with congenital glaucoma. The eye has been subjected to several sclerectomies. Extensive visual field defects are evident in both types of test results.

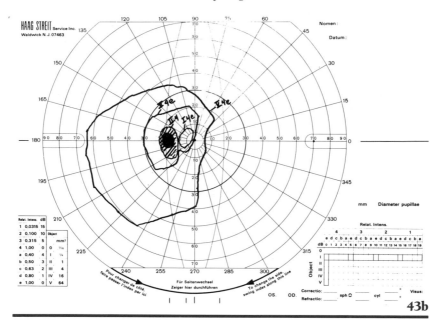

Shallow defects detected by manual kinetic perimetry are generally carefully investigated and are considered to be true defects only when they are well-defined. The larger and deeper the defect area, the more credible the results are considered to be. Similar requirements apply to test results from automatic static perimetry. Shallow 5 dB scotomata covering only one point, for example, regularly appear in normal fields simply because of the statistical uncertainties of the patient's responses (Wilensky and Joondeph 1984). Common sense demands that such a shallow defect extend over a number of tested points in order to be considered a true defect. If the disturbance involves two or three points in the same area, points which follow a logical pattern, then there may be cause for concern.

If a questionable area is small or shallow or otherwise not absolutely obvious on the grayscale printout, look at the defect depth printout of threshold results to see how many points have caused the disturbance. It will show the number of disturbed points and the extent of departure of each from the expected value. The numeric printout (lower right third of a three-in-one printout) makes even more precise analysis possible. In this presentation of test results, the threshold level at each point may be compared with that of the surrounding points and with its mirror image points in the other quadrants.

Field defects that would be evident with older perimetric techniques will show up very clearly in computerized perimetry (figure 44). It should be remembered that the automatic instruments test in a highly sophisticated, consistent and objective manner, and as a result, they will often find field defects which may have been missed by manual kinetic techniques.

**Figure 44.** This 46-year-old male patient was referred because of subjective deterioration of vision. Visual acuity was 20/20 in the right eye and 20/20-25 in the left eye with spectacle correction. Fundus examination showed somewhat blurred, slightly pale discs with irregular demarcation and mostly buried drusen. The diagnosis was optic nerve drusen. The visual fields are clearly pathological in both eyes.

Note that the defects as shown in the Field Analyzer results are deeper than those found with kinetic perimetry. For example, at about 30° infero-temporally in the Humphrey results for the right eye, the patient was unable to see static stimuli equivalent to a Goldmann V4e. In that same area on the Goldmann results, the patient was able to see a II4e kinetic stimulus, a difference of about 1.5 log units from the static results.

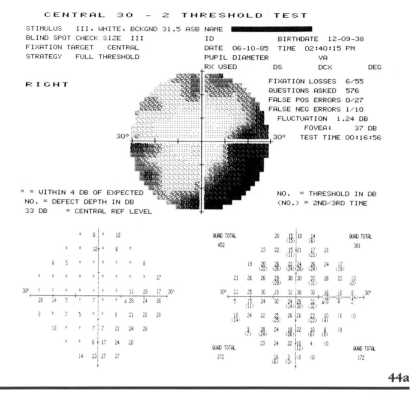

CENTRAL 30 - 2 THRESHOLD TEST

STIMULUS   III, WHITE, BCKGND 31.5 ASB NAME ▮▮▮▮▮▮▮▮▮▮▮
BLIND SPOT CHECK SIZE III              ID              BIRTHDATE  12-09-38
FIXATION TARGET   CENTRAL              DATE  06-10-85  TIME  02:40:15 PM
STRATEGY   FULL THRESHOLD             PUPIL DIAMETER        VA
                                      RX USED      DS      DCX        DEG

RIGHT                                 FIXATION LOSSES  6/55
                                      QUESTIONS ASKED  576
                                      FALSE POS ERRORS 0/27
                                      FALSE NEG ERRORS 1/10
                                      FLUCTUATION  1.24 DB
                                              FOVEA:      37 DB
          30°                    30°   TEST TIME 00:16:56

◇ = WITHIN 4 DB OF EXPECTED                  NO.  = THRESHOLD IN DB
NO. = DEFECT DEPTH IN DB                     (NO.) = 2ND/3RD TIME
33 DB  = CENTRAL REF LEVEL

**44a**

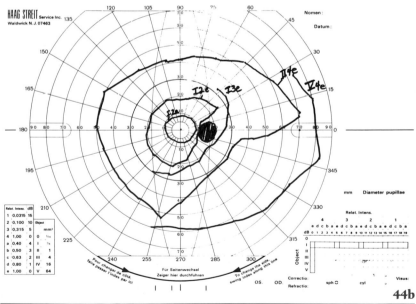

**44b**

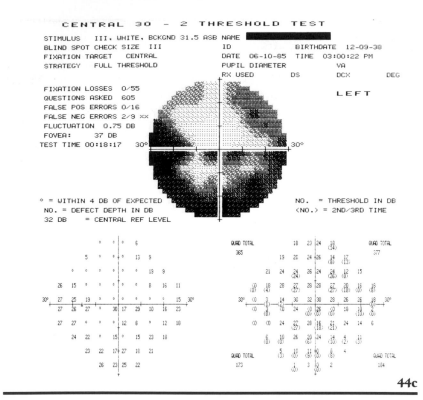

### CENTRAL 30 - 2 THRESHOLD TEST

STIMULUS    III, WHITE, BCKGND 31.5 ASB NAME ▮▮▮▮▮▮▮
BLIND SPOT CHECK SIZE  III              ID                BIRTHDATE  12-09-38
FIXATION TARGET    CENTRAL              DATE  06-10-85  TIME  03:00:22 PM
STRATEGY    FULL THRESHOLD             PUPIL DIAMETER             VA
                                       RX USED        DS     DCX      DEG

FIXATION LOSSES  0/55                                      LEFT
QUESTIONS ASKED  605
FALSE POS ERRORS 0/16
FALSE NEG ERRORS 2/9 xx
FLUCTUATION  0.75 DB
FOVEA:      37 DB
TEST TIME 00:18:17     30°                        30°

° = WITHIN 4 DB OF EXPECTED                    NO.  = THRESHOLD IN DB
NO. = DEFECT DEPTH IN DB                       (NO.) = 2ND/3RD TIME
32 DB   = CENTRAL REF LEVEL

**44c**

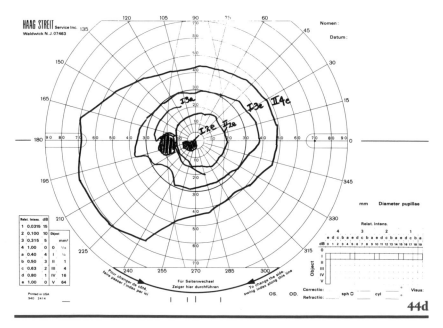

**44d**

# GLAUCOMA

**T**HE CURRENTLY accepted definition of glaucomatous field loss is that in the early stages there are small areas of depressed sensitivity in the Bjerrum area. These depressed areas are more common on the nasal side. Later they enlarge and develop into the full-blown arcuate Bjerrum defect (figure 45). They are more often found superiorly (figure 46), and nasal steps are very common (figure 47). Figure 48 illustrates another example of well-developed glaucoma, in this case with a double arcuate defect.

Notice that nowhere in the above description is enlargement of the blind spot discussed. It was once thought that such enlargement was one of the primary signs of early glaucoma. However, over the past twenty years, several researchers, beginning with Aulhorn and Harms in 1966, have documented the development of glaucoma summarized in the foregoing paragraph, and nowhere has it been shown that the blind spot enlarges (Aulhorn and Harms 1967; Drance, Wheeler and Patullo 1967; Drance 1969; LeBlanc and Becker 1971; Werner and Drance 1977; Heijl and Lundqvist 1983).

The view that enlarged blind spots indicate glaucoma may have arisen for two reasons. First, arcuate scotomata are sometimes located adjacent to the blind spot; this is not the most common place for early field loss, but it does happen. Obviously, this could be called an enlarged blind spot, but it is not what was originally meant by saying that blind spot enlargement is an early sign of glaucoma (figure 49). Second, it is quite probable that enlarged blind spots are found more often in glaucomatous than in normal fields because peripapillary atrophies are more common in glaucoma patients than in normals. It is unlikely that such an enlarged blind spot would follow or be caused by the glaucoma; nor is it likely that it would become larger as the disease progressed, as peripapillary atrophies are generally stable and non-pathological.

Before clear-cut glaucomatous field defects develop, there is a stage, often several years long, during which field defects come and go in the area which later becomes definitely pathological. This has been established retrospectively (Werner and Drance 1977). In fact, the most typical thing about very early glaucomatous field loss is its variability, or fluctuation, within a single test session and from session to session. Therefore, because perimetric results are so variable in the early stages of the disease, it can be impossible to tell from any one test that the disease is present. Unstable areas should be watched carefully (figure 50). In some cases, of course, the disease does seem to progress steadily over a relatively short period of time (figure 51).

**Figure 45.** Five stages of the development of glaucomatous field loss (Aulhorn 1978). In stage 1, relative defects are seen in the arcuate area. In kinetic perimetry results, these are most often seen as constrictions of the isopters in the range of 5° to 25° from fixation. In static threshold perimetry results, they may be seen as variable small scotomata in the same areas.

Stage 2 shows spot-like deep defects, or scotomata, still not connected with the blind spot. Note that in both stage one and two, field loss is most often seen in the nasal field, and is seldom manifested as an enlargement of the blind spot.

Stage 3 shows an arcuate scotoma, often with breakthrough into the nasal periphery, producing a classical nasal step.

Stage 4 defects may show extensive ring or half ring scotomata, leaving a central island of vision, as well as peripheral vision.

In stage 5, the central hill of vision has usually collapsed, leaving only the temporal visual field.

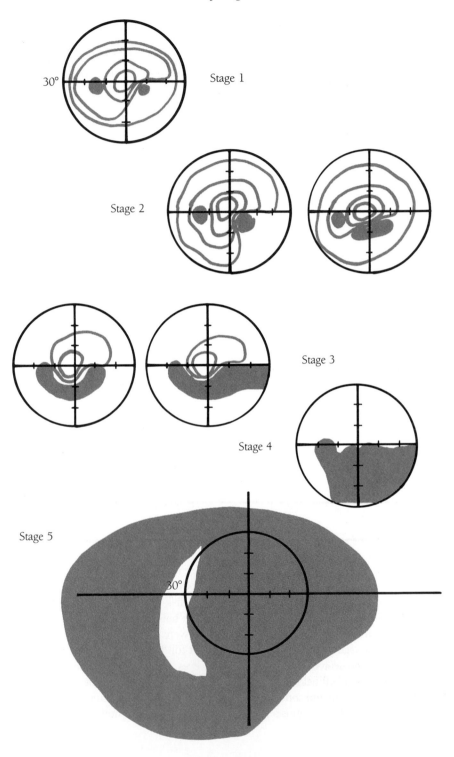

Stage 1

Stage 2

Stage 3

Stage 4

Stage 5

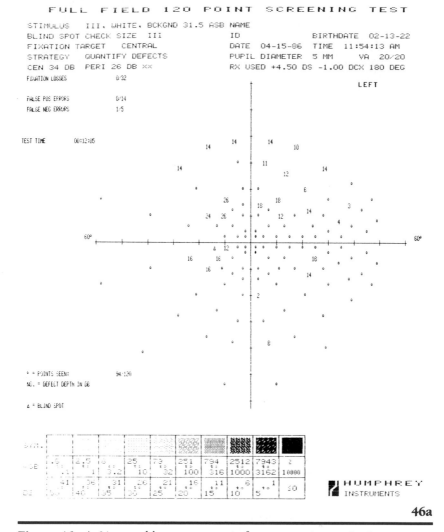

**Figure 46.** A 64-year-old woman came in for optometric examination complaining of blur when reading. This was remedied with a change in her refractive correction. Fundus examination showed extensive asymmetric deep cupping of the optic nerves, with cup to disk ratios of 0.75/0.85 OD, and 0.50/0.55 OS (horizontal/vertical). Applanation tensions were OD 14 and OS 13. External and slit lamp biomicroscopy were unremarkable.

Perimetric examination using the 120-point full field screening test showed numerous deep scotomata centrally in both eyes, and extensive losses in the peripiheral nasal field in the right eye. Repeat examination one week later confirmed the field and tonometric findings, and medical consultation was recommended. The diagnosis was low tension glaucoma, and the patient is being followed.

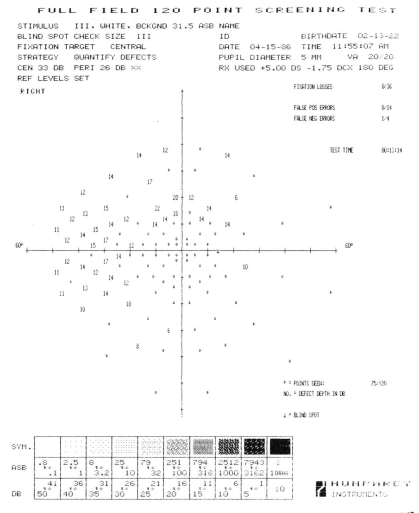

FULL FIELD 120 POINT SCREENING TEST

STIMULUS    III. WHITE. BCKGND 31.5 ASB NAME
BLIND SPOT CHECK SIZE   III                    ID          BIRTHDATE  02-13-22
FIXATION TARGET   CENTRAL                       DATE  04-15-86  TIME  11:55:07 AM
STRATEGY   QUANTIFY DEFECTS                      PUPIL DIAMETER  5 MM      VA  20/20
CEN 33 DB   PERI 26 DB ××                        RX USED +5.00 DS -1.75 DCX 180 DEG
REF LEVELS SET

RIGHT

FIXATION LOSSES        0/36
FALSE POS ERRORS       0/14
FALSE NEG ERRORS       1/4

TEST TIME        00:13:14

° = POINTS SEEN:          75/120
NO. = DEFECT DEPTH IN DB

△ = BLIND SPOT

| SYM. | | | | | | | | | | |
|------|----|----|----|----|----|----|----|----|----|----|
| ASB | .8 to .1 | 2.5 to 1 | 8 to 3.2 | 25 to 10 | 79 to 32 | 251 to 100 | 794 to 316 | 2512 to 1000 | 7943 to 3162 | 2 10000 |
| DB | 41 to 50 | 36 to 40 | 31 to 35 | 26 to 30 | 21 to 25 | 16 to 20 | 11 to 15 | 6 to 10 | 1 to 5 | ≤0 |

HUMPHREY
INSTRUMENTS

**46b**

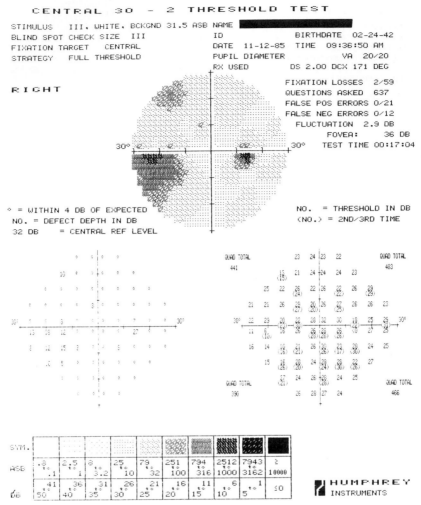

**Figure 47.** This field shows the classical nasal step pattern often seen in glaucoma patients. The patient is a 42-year-old man with a diagnosis of pigment dispersion glaucoma, pressures of OD 39 and OS 25, and cup to disk ratios of approximately OD 0.7 and OS 0.6. As the results of the 30-2 threshold test show, there has been significant loss of sensitivity in the central nasal field below the horizontal meridian. Note also the three relative scotomata in the arcuate area, two in the superior nasal field, and one in the infero-temporal field. Significant nasal steps may be accompanied by shallow transient losses elsewhere in the central and/or peripheral fields.

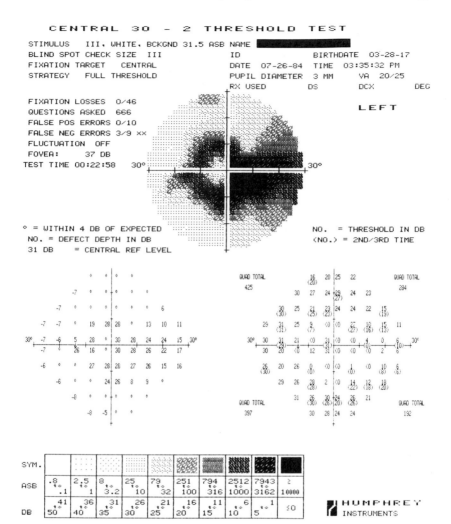

**Figure 48.** A central 30-2 threshold test run on the left eye of a 67-year-old woman shows well-developed double arcuate defects. The patient has a history of glaucoma and cataracts. Intraocular pressure was 19 mmHg under maximal medication. Notching was observed at 6:00 and 12:00. Cup to disc ratio was 0.5 x 0.7.

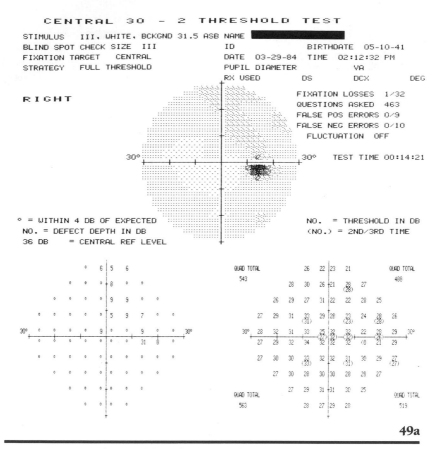

CENTRAL 30 - 2 THRESHOLD TEST

STIMULUS   III, WHITE, BCKGND 31.5 ASB NAME ████████████████
BLIND SPOT CHECK SIZE  III                  ID                    BIRTHDATE  05-10-41
FIXATION TARGET    CENTRAL                  DATE   03-29-84  TIME  02:12:32 PM
STRATEGY   FULL THRESHOLD                   PUPIL DIAMETER              VA
                                            RX USED        DS      DCX        DEG

RIGHT                                       FIXATION LOSSES   1/32
                                            QUESTIONS ASKED   463
                                            FALSE POS ERRORS  0/9
                                            FALSE NEG ERRORS  0/10
                                               FLUCTUATION  OFF

               30°                      30°    TEST TIME 00:14:21

° = WITHIN 4 DB OF EXPECTED                    NO.  = THRESHOLD IN DB
NO. = DEFECT DEPTH IN DB                      (NO.) = 2ND/3RD TIME
36 DB   = CENTRAL REF LEVEL

**Figure 49.** Humphrey Field Analyzer central 30-2 threshold tests were run nine months apart on the right eye of a 43-year-old man with pigmentary glaucoma. Note that the blind spot has not enlarged, but rather, a Bjerrum scotoma has developed adjacent to it. Increased intraocular pressures (OD 30-39 and OS 25-28) and pigment dispersion syndromes had been found in 1981. The discs were, and still are, tilted, myopic with a conus and without distinct glaucomatous signs. The patient received a pilocarpine insert and later timolol maleate, but the pressure in the right eye was only reduced to 26-30 mmHg.

When the first 30-2 test shown here was run on the right eye in 1984 (figure 49a), there was a suspicion of field defects. The patient underwent laser trabeculoplasty twice, but the pressure remained in the mid 20s. The second 30-2 test shown here (figure 49b) revealed more distinct field defects, and the patient was subjected to trabeculectomy. The intraocular pressure is now 17 mmHg, and best corrected visual acuity is 20/20.

Statpac single field analyses of these test results can be seen in figure 75 in chapter 6.

# CENTRAL 30 - 2 THRESHOLD TEST

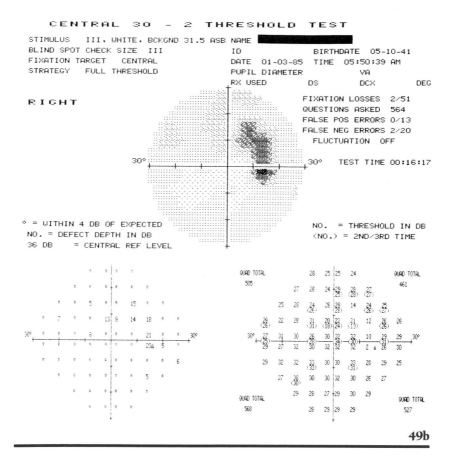

STIMULUS    III, WHITE, BCKGND 31.5 ASB   NAME ████████████

BLIND SPOT CHECK SIZE   III
FIXATION TARGET    CENTRAL
STRATEGY    FULL THRESHOLD

ID                           BIRTHDATE   05-10-41
DATE   01-03-85   TIME   05:50:39 AM
PUPIL DIAMETER                VA
RX USED           DS          DCX          DEG

RIGHT

FIXATION LOSSES   2/51
QUESTIONS ASKED   564
FALSE POS ERRORS 0/13
FALSE NEG ERRORS 2/20
   FLUCTUATION  OFF

30°                                    30°   TEST TIME 00:16:17

° = WITHIN 4 DB OF EXPECTED
NO. = DEFECT DEPTH IN DB
36 DB   = CENTRAL REF LEVEL

NO.  = THRESHOLD IN DB
(NO.) = 2ND/3RD TIME

**49b**

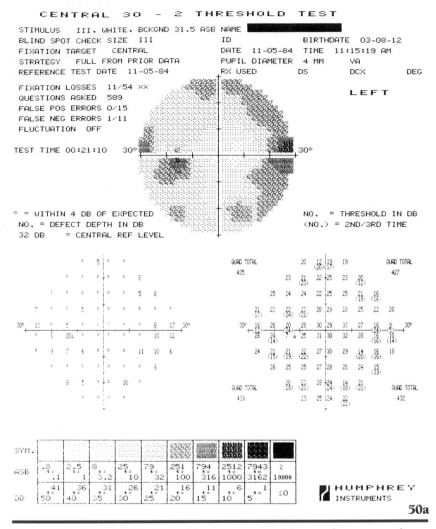

**Figure 50.** Central 30-2 threshold tests were run eight months apart on the left eye of a 72-year-old woman suspected of having glaucoma. What appear to be clear visual field defects in the November 1984 test (figure 50a) are not present in February 1985 test results (figure 50b).

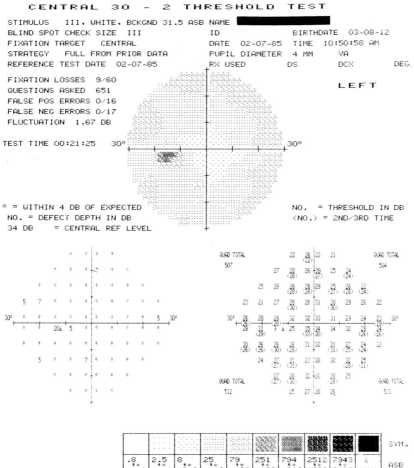

CENTRAL 30 - 2 THRESHOLD TEST

STIMULUS    III. WHITE. BCKGND 31.5 ASB NAME ▓▓▓▓▓
BLIND SPOT CHECK SIZE   III          ID                    BIRTHDATE   03-08-12
FIXATION TARGET   CENTRAL            DATE   02-07-85   TIME  10:50:58 AM
STRATEGY    FULL FROM PRIOR DATA     PUPIL DIAMETER   4 MM       VA
REFERENCE TEST DATE  02-07-85        RX USED          DS         DCX         DEG.

FIXATION LOSSES   9/60
QUESTIONS ASKED   651                                          LEFT
FALSE POS ERRORS 0/16
FALSE NEG ERRORS 0/17
FLUCTUATION   1.67 DB

TEST TIME 00:21:25    30°                                30°

° = WITHIN 4 DB OF EXPECTED                    NO.  = THRESHOLD IN DB
NO. = DEFECT DEPTH IN DB                       (NO.) = 2ND/3RD TIME
34 DB    = CENTRAL REF LEVEL

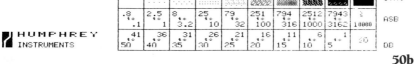

HUMPHREY
INSTRUMENTS

**50b**

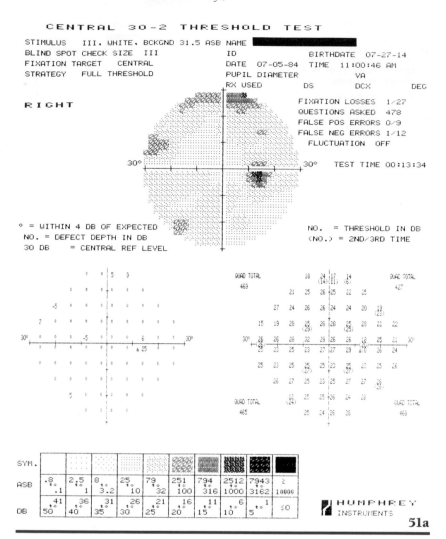

**Figure 51.** Over the course of eight months, a series of four central 30-2 threshold tests was run on the right eye of a 70-year-old woman whose intraocular pressures had been known to be increased for at least ten years. She had been followed for many years with no medication while the pressures remained in the 20s. There was progressive cupping of the right disc and intolerance to pilocarpine, epinephrine and timolol maleate. Testing showed the visual field normal up to July, 1984 (figure 51a). Three central 30-2 threshold tests taken between November 1984 and March 1985 (figures 51b, 51c and 51d) show definite, and probably progressive, inferior nasal field defects. The right disc shows vertically elongated cupping, oddly enough with the thinnest rim inferiorly. The right eye was subjected to laser trabeculoplasty in April 1985 with a resulting pressure reduction to 11 mmHg.

Statpac analyses of these test results and of two subsequent follow-up tests are shown in figure 81 in chapter 6.

# CENTRAL 30 - 2 THRESHOLD TEST

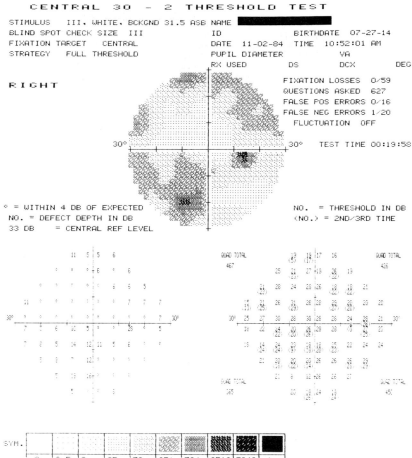

STIMULUS   III. WHITE. BCKGND 31.5 ASB  NAME ████████████
BLIND SPOT CHECK SIZE   III                    ID                    BIRTHDATE  07-27-14
FIXATION TARGET    CENTRAL                     DATE   11-02-84   TIME   10:52:01 AM
STRATEGY    FULL THRESHOLD                     PUPIL DIAMETER              VA
                                               RX USED            DS        DCX          DEG

RIGHT                                          FIXATION LOSSES   0/59
                                               QUESTIONS ASKED   627
                                               FALSE POS ERRORS  0/16
                                               FALSE NEG ERRORS  1/20
                                                FLUCTUATION   OFF

           30°                          30°    TEST TIME 00:19:58

° = WITHIN 4 DB OF EXPECTED                    NO.  = THRESHOLD IN DB
NO. = DEFECT DEPTH IN DB                       (NO.) = 2ND/3RD TIME
33 DB    = CENTRAL REF LEVEL

| SYM. | | | | | | | | | | | |
|---|---|---|---|---|---|---|---|---|---|---|---|
| ASB | .8 to .1 | 2.5 to 1 | 8 to 3.2 | 25 to 10 | 79 to 32 | 251 to 100 | 794 to 316 | 2512 to 1000 | 7943 to 3162 | 2 to 10000 | |
| DB | 41 to 50 | 36 to 40 | 31 to 35 | 26 to 30 | 21 to 25 | 16 to 20 | 11 to 15 | 6 to 10 | 1 to 5 | ≤0 | |

**HUMPHREY** INSTRUMENTS

**51b**

CENTRAL 30 - 2 THRESHOLD TEST

STIMULUS   III, WHITE, BCKGND 31.5 ASB NAME ▮▮▮▮▮▮▮▮
BLIND SPOT CHECK SIZE   III          ID                  BIRTHDATE  07-27-14
FIXATION TARGET    CENTRAL           DATE  11-22-84  TIME  08:33:28 AM
STRATEGY   FULL THRESHOLD            PUPIL DIAMETER              VA
                                     RX USED         DS      DCX        DEG

RIGHT                                          FIXATION LOSSES  1/52
                                               QUESTIONS ASKED  562
                                               FALSE POS ERRORS 0/10
                                               FALSE NEG ERRORS 2/19
                                                  FLUCTUATION  2.32 DB

          30°                            30°   TEST TIME 00:18:13

° = WITHIN 4 DB OF EXPECTED               NO.  = THRESHOLD IN DB
NO. = DEFECT DEPTH IN DB                 (NO.) = 2ND/3RD TIME
34 DB   = CENTRAL REF LEVEL

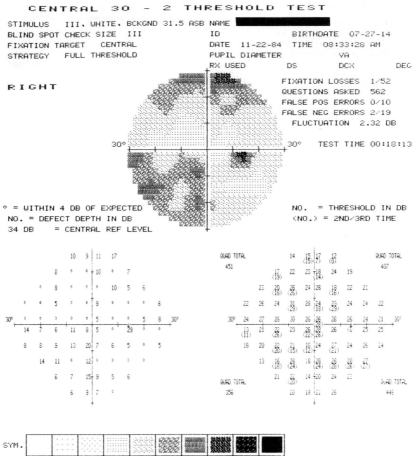

| SYM. | | | | | | | | | | |
|---|---|---|---|---|---|---|---|---|---|---|
| ASB | .8 to .1 | 2.5 to 1 | 8 to 3.2 | 25 to 10 | 79 to 32 | 251 to 100 | 794 to 316 | 2512 to 1000 | 7943 to 3162 | ≥ 10000 |
| DB | 41 to 50 | 36 to 40 | 31 to 35 | 26 to 30 | 21 to 25 | 16 to 20 | 11 to 15 | 6 to 10 | 1 to 5 | ≤0 |

HUMPHREY INSTRUMENTS

**51c**

# CENTRAL 30 - 2 THRESHOLD TEST

STIMULUS   III, WHITE, BCKGND 31.5 ASB NAME ███████████
BLIND SPOT CHECK SIZE   III                ID                    BIRTHDATE  07-27-14
FIXATION TARGET    CENTRAL                 DATE  03-08-85  TIME  08:55:51 AM
STRATEGY    FULL THRESHOLD                 PUPIL DIAMETER            VA
                                           RX USED        DS        DCX        DEG

RIGHT

FIXATION LOSSES   0/59
QUESTIONS ASKED   621
FALSE POS ERRORS  0/24
FALSE NEG ERRORS  0/13
 FLUCTUATION   2.05 DB

30°                                        30°   TEST TIME 00:19:05

° = WITHIN 4 DB OF EXPECTED                NO.  = THRESHOLD IN DB
NO. = DEFECT DEPTH IN DB                   (NO.) = 2ND/3RD TIME
30 DB   = CENTRAL REF LEVEL

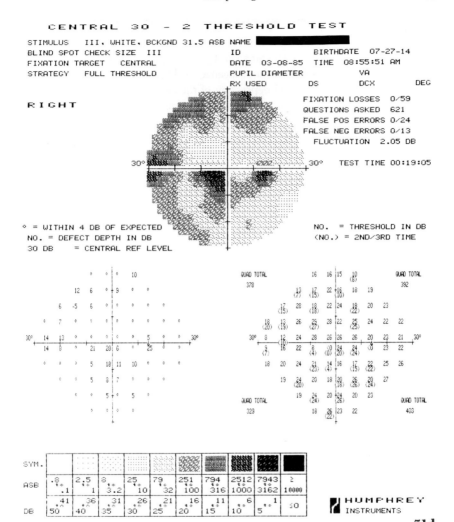

SYM.

| ASB | .8 to .1 | 2.5 to 1 | 8 to 3.2 | 25 to 10 | 79 to 32 | 251 to 100 | 794 to 316 | 2512 to 1000 | 7943 to 3162 | ≥ 10000 |
|---|---|---|---|---|---|---|---|---|---|---|
| DB | 41 to 50 | 36 to 40 | 31 to 35 | 26 to 30 | 21 to 25 | 16 to 20 | 11 to 15 | 6 to 10 | 1 to 5 | ≤0 |

HUMPHREY
INSTRUMENTS

**51d**

## Overall Depression

Glaucoma can lead to a general depression of the field without localized field defects. However, an overall depression of the field is such a general sign that it usually lacks diagnostic value in an individual patient.

As described earlier, each Field Analyzer test result printout includes an index called the central reference level, which helps the practitioner determine whether or not there is an overall depression. This index indicates the overall height of the patient's hill of vision, which varies in the normal population as a function of age, testing experience, media clarity, refraction, and other factors.

General depression is often a sign of media opacities, especially if the patient also has small pupils. With an inexperienced perimetric subject, test results sometimes show a general depression of sensitivity which disappears with training. Poor patient alertness can also produce test results that suggest general depression. In some cases, inappropriate refractive correction can give the impression of overall field loss (see figure 71, page 126), but using a size III stimulus or larger should minimize poor refraction as a source of overall depression (Sloan 1961; Benedetto and Cyrlin 1985).

The most that should be said is that general depression is more common in groups of patients who have already been identified as glaucoma suspects by questionable or pathological disks but who show no localized field loss (Flammer, Eppler and Niesel 1982). When a very clear, repeatable test result showing overall field loss occurs, it is important to take the time to find out the cause.

## Following Up Glaucoma

With a disease such as glaucoma, which progresses slowly, it is generally very difficult to establish whether a patient's condition is stable or deteriorating by using only two or three field tests. It is hard to differentiate between normal variation caused by physiologic variation or increased variation caused by disease; the zone of uncertainty is large. It is fairly certain that a field defect has progressed if it can be shown at least twice that it covers an area which has not been afflicted previously. That often means it is necessary to take a minimum of four tests (two tests to establish a baseline and two tests for follow-up).

Whenever a field defect looks definitely larger over time, check to see whether fixation has improved. In such cases, any field defects will show up more clearly. If one test shows very poor fixation and a certain size field defect, and the next test shows much better fixation, the field defect will tend to look larger and stand out more clearly even if no real physiological change has taken place. That should be taken into account in following up a field and not be mistaken for deterioration. It should also be noted that many patients will improve their test performance as they acquire more experience with visual field testing (Aulhorn and Harms 1972). This factor should not be confused with true changes in the visual field.

The fluctuation measurements in the threshold test printouts can be helpful in follow-up testing because they provide an understanding of the amount of variability that is to be expected with an individual patient. There is a relationship between long-term stability and within-test stability. In general, the variability measured during a test predicts long-term variability fairly well (Bebie, Fankhauser and Spahr 1976). Take, for example, a patient who has a field defect that shows up on the test reproducibly and who also has a fairly low fluctuation, say 2 db or so. It does not require as much change in the field in such a case to suggest the disease is progressing as it would with a patient who has a very high fluctuation value.

It should be remembered that when a follow-up test is run with the fast-threshold strategy, which tests points at 2 dB brighter than the values found on the previous test, normal variation can be so large that points will be missed at plus 2 dB even if no progression has taken place.

# NEUROLOGICAL DISEASE

**E** VALUATION OF the visual field is particularly
important in neuro-ophthalmological examination. The pattern of visual field loss can indicate
very precisely which portions of the visual system are
involved, especially when the visual fields of the
two eyes are compared.

Neuro-ophthalmological visual field defects may be
due to lesions of the optic nerve, optic chiasm, or
post chiasmal structures. Optic nerve lesions produce
either central or nerve fiber bundle type field
defects, only in the affected eye. A unilateral central
scotoma is most likely due to optic neuritis (figure 52)
or a compressive lesion. Nerve fiber bundle defects
similar to those seen in glaucoma may be caused by
optic nerve drusen (refer back to figure 44, page
64), chronic papilledema, or ischemic optic neuropathy
(figure 53).

Optic nerve fibers from the nasal retina cross in the
optic chiasm with the most inferior nasal fibers
crossing first. These fibers pass slightly forward in the
contralateral optic nerve (Willebrandt's knee) prior
to continuing their posterior course. Thus, a mass in
the posterior optic nerve may produce a central
scotoma ipsilaterally and a superior temporal field
defect in the contralateral eye (figure 54).

Lesions at the optic chiasm produce bitemporal
visual field defects that tend to obey the vertical
meridian. Thus, the classical field finding in pituitary
adenoma is a marked loss of much of the left field
in the left eye, and similar loss of much of the right
field in the right eye (figure 55).

In contrast to optic chiasm disease, lesions involving
structures posterior to the chiasm produce the same
or similar field defects in both eyes, and the more
posterior the lesion the more similar the defects will
be. Here again field loss will tend to obey the vertical
meridian, and thus will probably involve either the
right or the left field of both eyes. Hence, a homonymous hemianopia may occur with a lesion in the
optic tract, lateral geniculate body, optic radiations

(figure 56), or occipital lobe (figures 57 and 58). Lesions of the occipital lobe produce extremely congruous visual field defects, i.e., the defects are very similar in the two eyes. The macular or extreme temporal visual fields may be spared in occipital disease, this being unique to defects localized in this region (figure 59).

Multiple sclerosis may produce variable field loss (figure 60). Congenital anomalies (figure 61) can cause field loss in apparently healthy patients. (See also figure 62.)

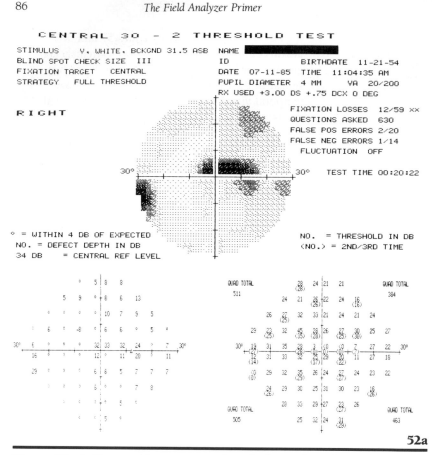

**52a**

**Figure 52.** A 32-year-old woman complained of acute loss of central vision in the right eye. In addition, the patient noted pain behind the right eye with movement of the eyes. There were no other ocular or systemic complaints, and the previous medical history was unremarkable.

On examination, the visual acuity was 20/200 OD and 20/15 OS. During color vision testing, the patient got only the control plate on the right, and identified all of the color plates correctly with the left eye. A marked afferent pupillary defect was present on the right. Confrontation visual field testing revealed a dense central scotoma on the right. The funduscopic evaluation of both eyes was within normal limits.

A central 30-2 threshold test confirmed the presence of a dense central scotoma on the right eye (figure 52a). The visual field on the left eye was within normal limits. A diagnosis of retrobulbar optic neuritis was made. Over the next three weeks, the visual acuity in the right eye returned to normal. A central 30-2 threshold test taken at that time showed a normal field (figure 52b).

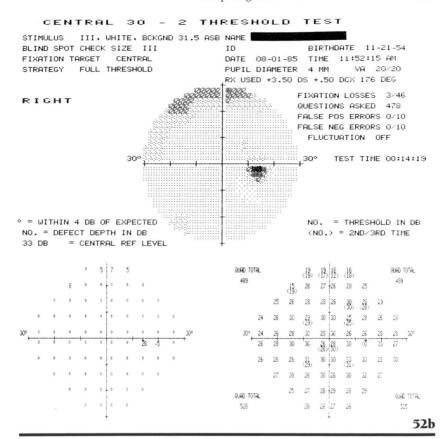

CENTRAL  30  -  2  THRESHOLD  TEST

STIMULUS    III. WHITE. BCKGND 31.5 ASB NAME
BLIND SPOT CHECK SIZE   III                    ID                    BIRTHDATE   11-21-54
FIXATION TARGET   CENTRAL                       DATE   08-01-85   TIME   11:52:15 AM
STRATEGY    FULL THRESHOLD                      PUPIL DIAMETER   4 MM      VA   20/20
                                                RX USED +3.50 DS +.50 DCX 176 DEG

RIGHT                                           FIXATION LOSSES   3/46
                                                QUESTIONS ASKED   478
                                                FALSE POS ERRORS 0/10
                                                FALSE NEG ERRORS 0/10
                                                   FLUCTUATION   OFF

30°                                        30°      TEST TIME 00:14:19

° = WITHIN 4 DB OF EXPECTED                     NO.  = THRESHOLD IN DB
NO. = DEFECT DEPTH IN DB                        (NO.) = 2ND/3RD TIME
33 DB    = CENTRAL REF LEVEL

**52b**

**Figure 53.** A 49-year-old man had awakened ten days previously with decreased vision in the lower half of the visual field of the right eye. This decrease in vision had remained unchanged. The vision in the left eye was normal. The previous ocular history was unremarkable. The patient suffered from mild hypertension that had been well controlled on medication. He denied any history of headache, fever, or other systemic symptoms.

On examination, the visual acuity with spectacle correction was 20/20 +2 OD and 20/15 OS. The patient was able to identify correctly seven out of eleven color plates with the right eye and all of the color plates with the left eye. Examination of the pupils revealed a mild afferent pupillary defect in the right eye. Funduscopy of the right eye revealed a moderate degree of disc edema, more marked superiorly than inferiorly. The remainder of the right fundus appeared normal. Examination of the disc on the left eye determined that no physiological cup was present. The remainder of the fundus examination was within normal limits. An erythrocyte sedimentation rate was 2.

A central 30-2 threshold test showed a dense inferior altitudinal visual field defect in the right eye. The visual field in the left eye was within normal limits. The diagnosis was idiopathic anterior ischemic optic neuropathy. The pattern of visual loss noted by the patient is characteristic for this disease. The absence of physiologic cupping of the left optic disc is suggestive of idiopathic anterior ischemic optic neuropathy as patients with this disorder often have no physiologic cup. Although a wide variety of visual field defects can be seen with anterior ischemic optic neuropathy, altitudinal defects are most common.

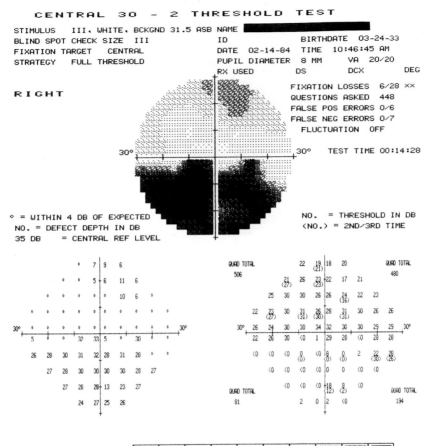

**CENTRAL 30 - 2 THRESHOLD TEST**

STIMULUS   III, WHITE, BCKGND 31.5 ASB  NAME ▮▮▮▮▮▮
BLIND SPOT CHECK SIZE  III          ID                    BIRTHDATE  03-24-33
FIXATION TARGET   CENTRAL           DATE  02-14-84  TIME   10:46:45 AM
STRATEGY   FULL THRESHOLD           PUPIL DIAMETER  8 MM        VA  20/20
                                    RX USED         DS        DCX          DEG

**RIGHT**

FIXATION LOSSES  6/28 ××
QUESTIONS ASKED  448
FALSE POS ERRORS 0/6
FALSE NEG ERRORS 0/7
   FLUCTUATION  OFF

30°                              30°   TEST TIME 00:14:28

○ = WITHIN 4 DB OF EXPECTED          NO.  = THRESHOLD IN DB
NO. = DEFECT DEPTH IN DB             ⟨NO.⟩ = 2ND/3RD TIME
35 DB  = CENTRAL REF LEVEL

**HUMPHREY INSTRUMENTS**

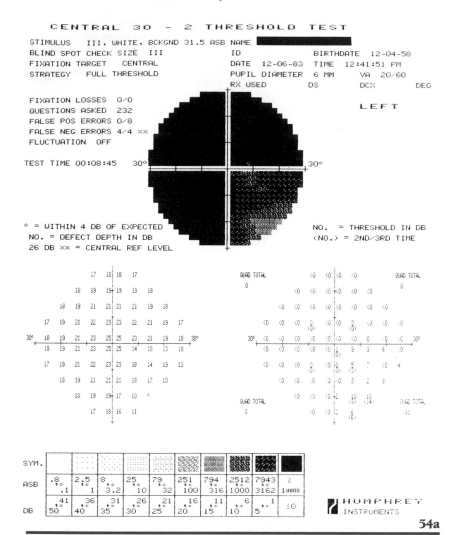

**Figure 54.** A 25-year-old man complained of progressive loss of vision in the left eye. The patient had no other ocular or systemic complaints.

Visual acuity was 20/20 OD and 20/60 OS without spectacle correction. During color vision testing the patient got all the plates correct on the right, but he correctly identified only the control plate with the left eye. Examination of the pupils determined the presence of a marked afferent pupillary defect on the left. Confrontation visual field testing revealed a central scotoma in the left eye. The remainder of a complete neuro-ophthalmologic examination was within normal limits.

A central 30-2 threshold test demonstrated almost total field loss in the central 30° of the left eye (figure 54a). A central 30-2 threshold test of the right eye revealed the presence of a superior temporal quadrant defect (figure 54b). With this finding, an immediate diagnosis of an anterior chiasmal

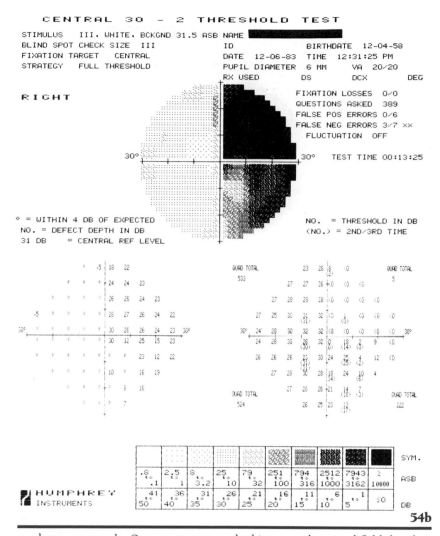

syndrome was made. One can assume on looking at such a visual field that the mass is compressing on the left optic nerve in addition to the anterior aspect of the chiasm. The fibers from the nasal retina cross in the optic chiasm with the most inferior nasal fibers crossing first. These fibers pass slightly forward in the contralateral optic nerve (Willebrant's knee) before continuing their posterior course. Hence, a mass in the posterior portion of the optic nerve will produce an ipsilateral central scotoma and a superior temporal field defect in the contralateral eye.

High resolution CT scanning of the head revealed extra-sellar extension of a pituitary tumor. The patient subsequently underwent transsphenoidal resection of a pituitary adenoma. He has remained stable for two years on hormonal replacement therapy.

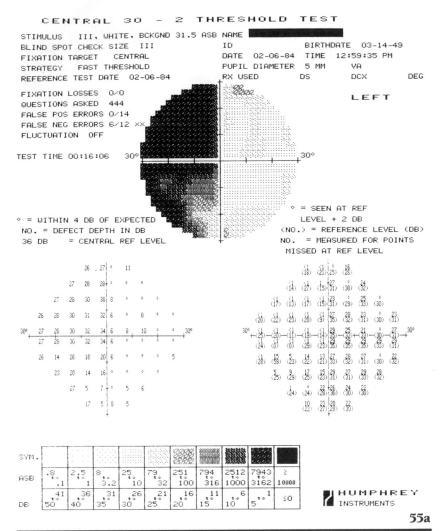

**Figure 55.** A 34-year-old woman was admitted to the hospital with her first episode of acute asthma. During a routine review of systems, the patient complained of amenorrhea and decreased libido since the age of twenty-two. The patient denied any visual or other systemic complaints.

An alert emergency room physician referred the patient for complete opthalmic examination. The visual acuity was 20/15 uncorrected. Color vision and pupillary light reflexes were normal. Central 30-2 threshold testing demonstrated a bitemporal hemianopia. A high-resolution CT scan of the head confirmed the presence of a pituitary adenoma. This was subsequently resected via a transsphenoidal approach.

# CENTRAL 30 — 2 THRESHOLD TEST

STIMULUS    III, WHITE, BCKGND 31.5 ASB   NAME ████████████
BLIND SPOT CHECK SIZE   III                        ID                    BIRTHDATE   03-14-49
FIXATION TARGET    CENTRAL                          DATE   02-06-84   TIME   12:39:34 PM
STRATEGY    FAST THRESHOLD                          PUPIL DIAMETER   5 MM   VA
REFERENCE TEST DATE   02-06-84                      RX USED          DS        DCX        DEG

RIGHT

FIXATION LOSSES   0/0
QUESTIONS ASKED   346
FALSE POS ERRORS  0/6
FALSE NEG ERRORS  2/10 XX
FLUCTUATION   OFF

30°                          30°   TEST TIME 00:12:28

° = WITHIN 4 DB OF EXPECTED
NO. = DEFECT DEPTH IN DB
37 DB    = CENTRAL REF LEVEL

° = SEEN AT REF
LEVEL + 2 DB
(NO.) = REFERENCE LEVEL (DB)
NO. = MEASURED FOR POINTS
MISSED AT REF LEVEL

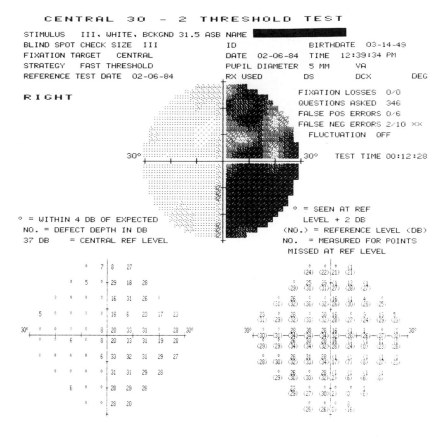

| SYM. | | | | | | | | | |
|---|---|---|---|---|---|---|---|---|---|
| ASB | .8 to .1 | 2.5 to 1 | 8 to 3.2 | 25 to 10 | 79 to 32 | 251 to 100 | 794 to 316 | 2512 to 1000 | 7943 to 3162 | ≥ 10000 |
| DB | 41 to 50 | 36 to 40 | 31 to 35 | 26 to 30 | 21 to 25 | 16 to 20 | 11 to 15 | 6 to 10 | 1 to 5 | ≤0 |

HUMPHREY
INSTRUMENTS

**55b**

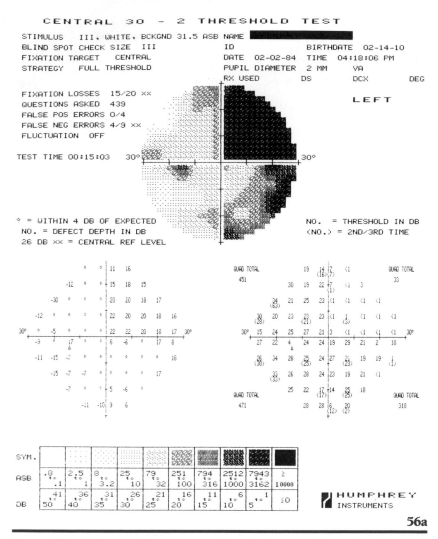

**Figure 56.** A 74-year-old woman complained of memory loss and confusion over a three- to four-month period. In addition, the patient complained of some difficulty seeing things out of the right eye. The previous ocular and medical histories were unremarkable.

Visual acuity in both eyes was 20/40. Color vision and pupillary light reflexes were normal. Slit lamp examination determined the presence of bilateral nuclear sclerotic cataracts. Funduscopy was unremarkable. Central 30-2 threshold testing revealed the presence of a right superior quadrantanopia in both eyes.

High-resolution CT scanning of the head showed a large left petrous ridge mass. A cerebral angiogram revealed the presence of tumor blush consistent with

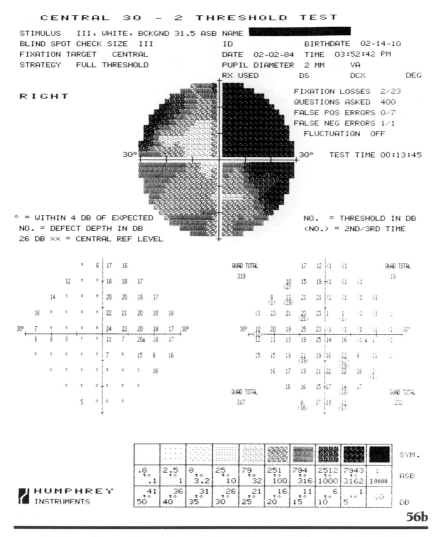

**56b**

a meningioma. The patient subsequently underwent a left temporal-parietal craniotomy with removal of a large meningioma attached to the tentorium petrous ridge.

Patients with homonymous visual field defects often complain, as this patient did, of visual loss in the eye contralateral to the lesion. In the elderly, these visual field defects are much more commonly due to ischemic cerebral events. However, adjuvant tests confirmed the presence of a meningioma in this case.

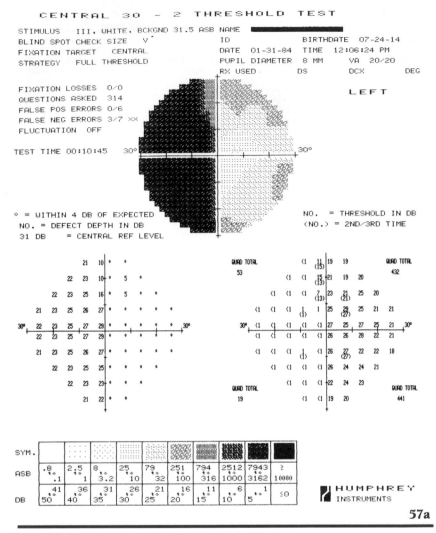

**Figure 57.** A 70-year-old woman suddenly developed a severe, throbbing holocranial headache while preparing lunch. The patient reported some "blurring" of the vision in both eyes and that the headache lasted all day. On awakening the following morning, she noted a loss of vision in the left eye. The previous ocular and medical histories were unremarkable.

On examination visual acuity was 20/20 OU with spectacle correction. The pupillary light reflexes were normal with no afferent pupillary defect. The remainder of a complete ophthalmic examination was within normal limits. The patient's pulse, however, was noted to be irregular.

A central 30-2 threshold test revealed the presence of a complete left homonymous hemianopia. An EKG confirmed the presence of atrial fibrillation. A high-resolution CT scan of the head revealed a right occipital lobe infarct.

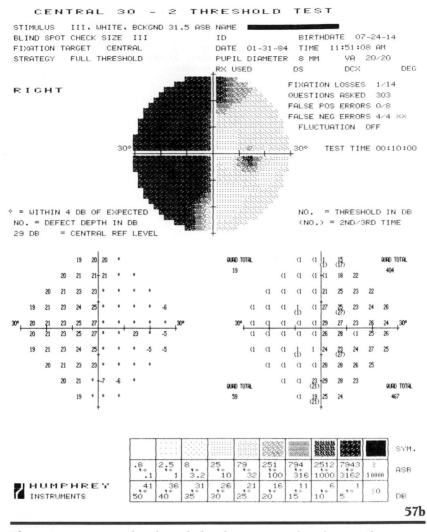

The patient was given digitalis and placed on anticoagulant therapy. She has remained stable for over a year.

The presence of a complete homonymous hemianopia is nonlocalizing. In this case, however, a high-resolution CT scan of the head was confirmatory for a right occipital lobe infarct. The presence of atrial fibrillation of recent onset made the diagnosis of embolic infarct of the right occipital lobe most likely.

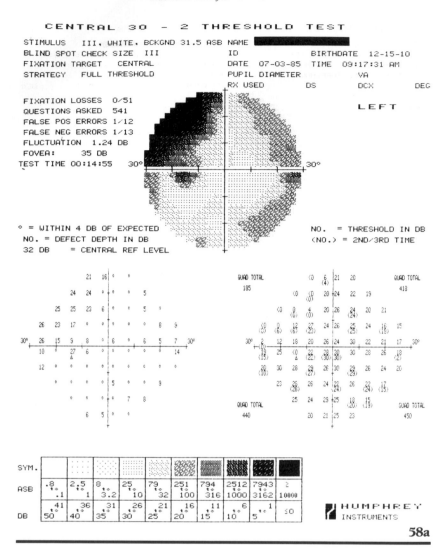

58a

**Figure 58.** This 75-year-old man had been followed for several years because of ocular hypertension (IOPs 23-41 mmHg). Discs were normal and acuity was 20/20 OU. Visual field testing every three months showed entirely normal fields up until September 1983, when rather congruous homonymous quadrantanopsias to the left were detected. The patient denied any neurological symptoms except an uncertain short attack of disorientation about one month earlier. CT scan showed a limited infarcture in the right temporal and occipital lobes. The visual field defects have remained stationary since then.

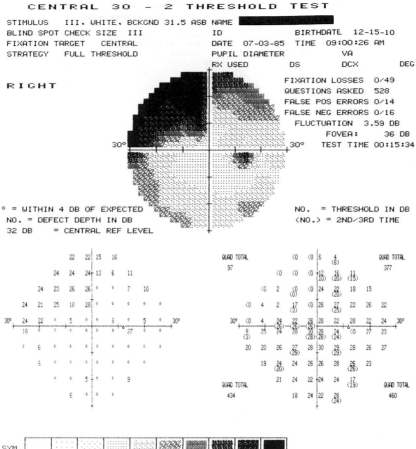

CENTRAL 30 - 2 THRESHOLD TEST

STIMULUS   III, WHITE, BCKGND 31.5 ASB NAME ▮▮▮▮▮▮▮▮▮▮▮
BLIND SPOT CHECK SIZE   III          ID                    BIRTHDATE   12-15-10
FIXATION TARGET   CENTRAL            DATE   07-03-85   TIME   09:00:26 AM
STRATEGY   FULL THRESHOLD           PUPIL DIAMETER              VA
                                     RX USED       DS        DCX         DEG

RIGHT

FIXATION LOSSES   0/49
QUESTIONS ASKED   528
FALSE POS ERRORS 0/14
FALSE NEG ERRORS 0/16
FLUCTUATION   3.59 DB
FOVEA:        36 DB
30°                                  30°   TEST TIME 00:15:34

° = WITHIN 4 DB OF EXPECTED                    NO.  = THRESHOLD IN DB
NO. = DEFECT DEPTH IN DB                       (NO.) = 2ND/3RD TIME
32 DB    = CENTRAL REF LEVEL

| SYM. | | | | | | | | | | |
|------|---|---|---|---|---|---|---|---|---|---|
| ASB | | .8 to .1 | 2.5 to 1 | 8 to 3.2 | 25 to 10 | 79 to 32 | 251 to 100 | 794 to 316 | 2512 to 1000 | 7943 to 3162 | ≥ 10000 |
| DB | 50 | 41 to 40 | 36 to 35 | 31 to 30 | 26 to 25 | 21 to 20 | 16 to 15 | 11 to 10 | 6 to 5 | 1 to | ≤0 |

HUMPHREY
INSTRUMENTS

**58b**

100        *The Field Analyzer Primer*

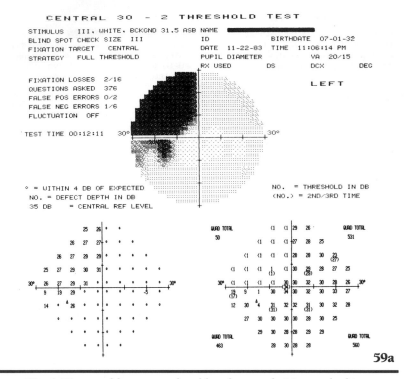

**Figure 59.** A 51-year-old man noted sudden decreased vision on looking to his left. His previous ocular history was unremarkable. The patient had noticed some shortness of breath over the past several weeks.

The visual acuity was 20/20 OD and 20/15 OS with spectacle correction. Confrontation visual field testing revealed the presence of a left superior quadrantanopia. A complete neuro-ophthalmological examination was otherwise within normal limits.

A central 30-2 threshold test confirmed the presence of the left superior quadrantanopia. In addition, a Field Analyzer temporal crescent threshold test revealed preservation of the left temporal crescent consistent with a lesion in the right occipital cortex. A high-resolution CT scan of the head confirmed this finding. On further evaluation, the patient was noted to have atrial fibrillation with a high ventricular rate. He was subsequently given digitalis and placed on anticoagulant therapy.

A crescent of temporal peripheral visual field is represented monocularly in the visual cortex. Preservation of the temporal crescent occurs occasionally with occipital lobe lesions only. The discovery of temporal crescent preservation in the left eye, as indicated by the temporal crescent threshold test (figure 59c), was diagnostic of an occipital lobe lesion as a cause for this patient's visual field defect.

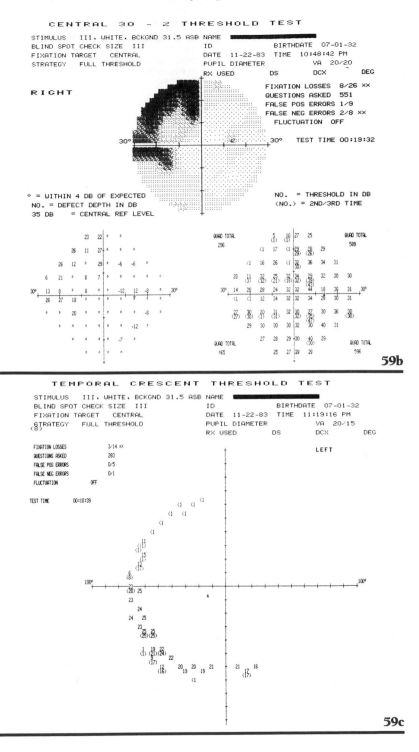

## CENTRAL 30 - 2 THRESHOLD TEST

STIMULUS   III, WHITE, BCKGND 31.5 ASB NAME ▬▬▬
BLIND SPOT CHECK SIZE  III                ID                    BIRTHDATE  07-01-32
FIXATION TARGET   CENTRAL                 DATE  11-22-83  TIME  10:48:42 PM
STRATEGY   FULL THRESHOLD                 PUPIL DIAMETER              VA  20/20
                                          RX USED        DS       DCX        DEG

**RIGHT**

FIXATION LOSSES   8/26 xx
QUESTIONS ASKED   551
FALSE POS ERRORS 1/9
FALSE NEG ERRORS 2/8 xx
FLUCTUATION   OFF

30°                                   30°    TEST TIME 00:19:32

° = WITHIN 4 DB OF EXPECTED               NO.  = THRESHOLD IN DB
NO. = DEFECT DEPTH IN DB                  <NO.> = 2ND/3RD TIME
35 DB  = CENTRAL REF LEVEL

**59b**

## TEMPORAL CRESCENT THRESHOLD TEST

STIMULUS   III, WHITE, BCKGND 31.5 ASB NAME ▬▬▬
BLIND SPOT CHECK SIZE  III                ID                    BIRTHDATE  07-01-32
FIXATION TARGET   CENTRAL                 DATE  11-22-83  TIME  11:19:16 PM
STRATEGY   FULL THRESHOLD                 PUPIL DIAMETER              VA  20/15
                                          RX USED        DS       DCX        DEG

FIXATION LOSSES         3/14 xx                                           LEFT
QUESTIONS ASKED         283
FALSE POS ERRORS        0/5
FALSE NEG ERRORS        0/1
FLUCTUATION       OFF

TEST TIME      00:10:39

100°                                                                      100°

**59c**

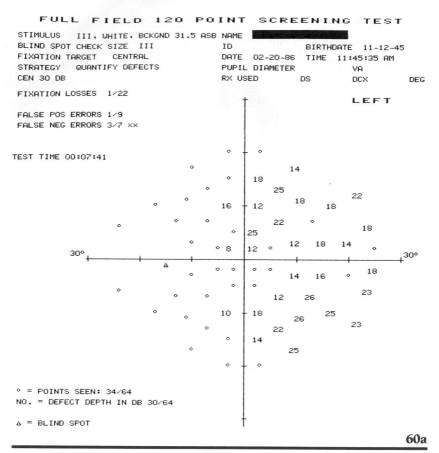

FULL FIELD 120 POINT SCREENING TEST

STIMULUS   III, WHITE, BCKGND 31.5 ASB  NAME  ████████████████
BLIND SPOT CHECK SIZE   III           ID                    BIRTHDATE  11-12-45
FIXATION TARGET   CENTRAL             DATE  02-20-86  TIME  11:45:35 AM
STRATEGY   QUANTIFY DEFECTS           PUPIL DIAMETER            VA
CEN 30 DB                             RX USED         DS       DCX        DEG

FIXATION LOSSES  1/22

FALSE POS ERRORS 1/9
FALSE NEG ERRORS 3/7 xx

TEST TIME 00:07:41

LEFT

30°                                                              30°

° = POINTS SEEN: 34/64
NO. = DEFECT DEPTH IN DB 30/64

△ = BLIND SPOT

**60a**

**Figure 60.** A 41-year-old male patient complained of difficulty with reading. Medical history revealed a recent diagnosis of multiple sclerosis. Screening with the central portion of the 120-point test showed dense homonymous field losses in both eyes. The patient was not aware of any field loss. All other eye findings were within expected limits, and simple presbyopic refractive correction remedied his presenting complaint.

A central scotoma has been reported to be the most common field defect in multiple sclerosis patients with visual complaints, although some researchers have found that the earliest defects in MS are isolated losses between 15 and 25 degrees from fixation. Defects may be highly variable with the exacerbations and remissions of the disease.

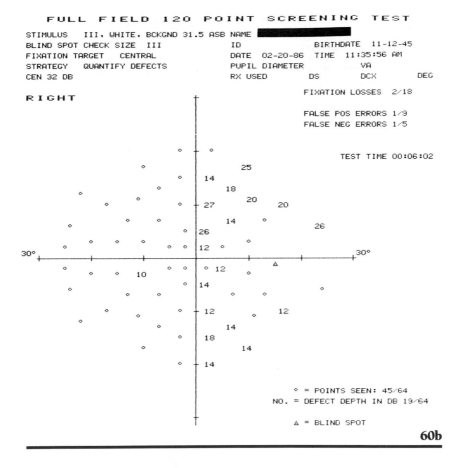

**60b**

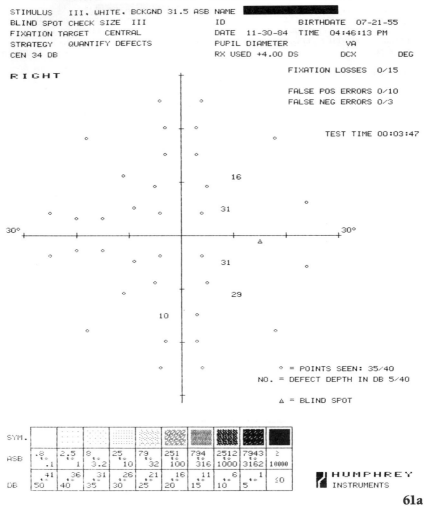

**Figure 61.** Routine field screening of a 29-year-old contact lens patient revealed a deep, large scotoma surrounding the blind spot in the right eye (figure 61a). Threshold testing with the 30-2 test pattern confirmed the finding (figure 61b). All other eye findings were unremarkable, except the observation of a congenitally abnormal disk, with a suggestion of drusen nasally and a large area of retinal pigment epithelial changes around the disk. Neuro-ophthalmological evaluation, fluorescein angiography, and electroretinography were all normal. Follow-up over a one-year period showed the field defect to be stable, and a diagnosis of congenital disk anomaly was made.

# CENTRAL 30 - 2 THRESHOLD TEST

STIMULUS   III, WHITE, BCKGND 31.5 ASB NAME ███████████
BLIND SPOT CHECK SIZE   OFF          ID                    BIRTHDATE   07-21-55
FIXATION TARGET   CENTRAL            DATE   11-30-84  TIME   05:30:07 PM
STRATEGY   FULL THRESHOLD           PUPIL DIAMETER              VA
                                    RX USED +4.00 DS       DCX           DEG

FIXATION LOSSES   0/0
QUESTIONS ASKED   509
FALSE POS ERRORS  0/20
FALSE NEG ERRORS  1/17
  FLUCTUATION   OFF

**RIGHT**

30°                                    30°        TEST TIME 00:12:59

∘ = WITHIN 4 DB OF EXPECTED                    NO.   = THRESHOLD IN DB
NO. = DEFECT DEPTH IN DB                      (NO.) = 2ND/3RD TIME
31 DB   = CENTRAL REF LEVEL

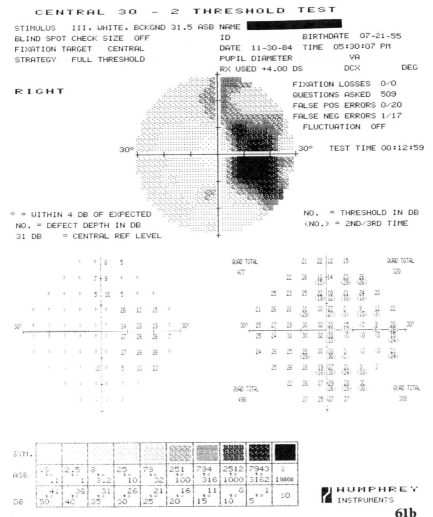

| SYM. | | | | | | | | | | |
|---|---|---|---|---|---|---|---|---|---|---|
| ASB | .3 to .1 | 2.5 to 1 | 8 to 3.2 | 25 to 10 | 79 to 32 | 251 to 100 | 794 to 316 | 2512 to 1000 | 7943 to 3162 | ≳ 10000 |
| DB | 41 to 50 | 36 to 40 | 31 to 35 | 26 to 30 | 21 to 25 | 16 to 20 | 11 to 15 | 6 to 10 | 1 to 5 | ≲0 |

◢ HUMPHREY
  INSTRUMENTS

**61b**

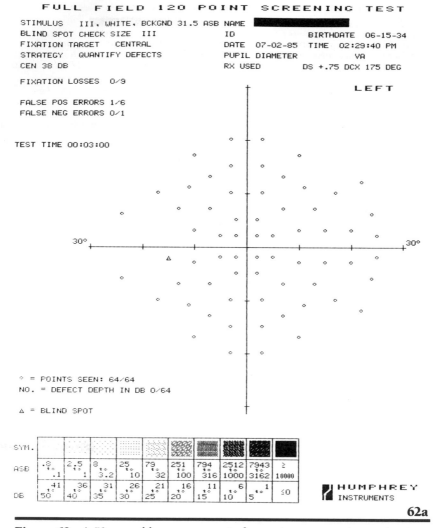

HUMPHREY
INSTRUMENTS

**Figure 62.** A 51-year-old woman came in for routine optometric examination. All aspects of her history and her examination findings were completely unremarkable, except for the results of a routine field screening.

The central portion of a Humphrey Field Analyzer full field 120-point screening test showed a normal visual field OS, but a markedly constricted field OD, to within 15 degrees of fixation (figure 62b). Fixation losses, and false positive and negative error checks all indicated that this was a highly reliable perimetry subject. Repeated screenings one week later confirmed the presence of field loss.

Neuro-ophthalmological evaluation showed no unusual findings. The patient refused a CT scan, and no cause for the lesion was discovered. The field was stable after one year.

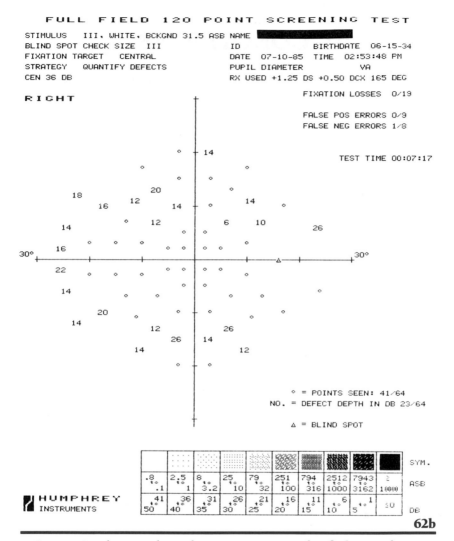

FULL FIELD 120 POINT SCREENING TEST

STIMULUS    III, WHITE, BCKGND 31.5 ASB NAME ▮▮▮▮▮▮▮▮▮▮▮▮
BLIND SPOT CHECK SIZE  III              ID                 BIRTHDATE  06-15-34
FIXATION TARGET    CENTRAL              DATE  07-10-85  TIME  02:53:48 PM
STRATEGY    QUANTIFY DEFECTS            PUPIL DIAMETER              VA
CEN 36 DB                              RX USED +1.25 DS +0.50 DCX 165 DEG

**RIGHT**

FIXATION LOSSES  0/19

FALSE POS ERRORS 0/9
FALSE NEG ERRORS 1/8

TEST TIME 00:07:17

° = POINTS SEEN: 41/64
NO. = DEFECT DEPTH IN DB 23/64

△ = BLIND SPOT

| | | | | | | | | | | SYM. |
|---|---|---|---|---|---|---|---|---|---|---|
| .8 to .1 | 2.5 to 1 | 8 to 3.2 | 25 to 10 | 79 to 32 | 251 to 100 | 794 to 316 | 2512 to 1000 | 7943 to 3162 | ≥ 10000 | ASB |
| 41 to 50 | 36 to 40 | 31 to 35 | 26 to 30 | 21 to 25 | 16 to 20 | 11 to 15 | 6 to 10 | 1 to 5 | ≤0 | DB |

**HUMPHREY**
INSTRUMENTS

**62b**

In screening the general population, it is not unusual to find cases of significant field loss which demand no medical intervention. In this case, the patient was asked to continue under medical supervision and advised about possible functional effects of her field loss.

# RETINAL CONDITIONS

**S** OMETIMES VISUAL field examination becomes important in the evaluation of a patient with retinal disease, or conversely, the results of the visual field examination may raise the possibility of a retinal diagnosis. Retinal diseases display characteristic visual field abnormalities. Findings may be unilateral or bilateral, depending on the underlying disease process. Retinal lesions usually produce absolute scotomata having discrete boundaries that correlate well with areas of retinal demise. Retinal diseases tend to produce scotomata which respect neither the vertical meridian nor the horizontal raphe. Despite these characteristics, visual field abnormalities arising from retinal lesions may sometimes mimic neurologic or glaucomatous processes.

Perhaps the most common type of retinal scotoma is the central scotoma of macular disease. This could be confused with the central scotoma of optic nerve disease or the paracentral scotomata of glaucoma (figures 63 and 64). Again, the retinal nature of the visual field abnormality is revealed by the discrete margins and density of the scotoma. Whether due to macular degeneration, central serous maculopathy, or other macular disease, lesions are usually bilateral, though they may be asymmetric. Ophthalmoscopy usually confirms the presence of macular diseases.

Occasionally, a retinal vascular lesion can produce a field defect which mimics that of optic nerve disease. Retinal branch artery and vein occlusions produce wedge-shaped infarctions of the retinal tissue they subserve, and wedge-shaped visual field defects result. If the occlusion is near the optic disc, the wedge may point toward the blind spot and resemble a nerve fiber bundle defect. If hemiretinal infarction occurs, the visual field defects may appear altitudinal (figure 65). These changes can usually be differentiated from true bundle defects by the absolute margins and wedge-shaped vs. arcuate morphology of the scotomata. Ophthalmoscopy will confirm the vascular occlusion.

Retinal detachments, whether rhegmatogenous or exudative, are somewhat of an exception to the rule. Unlike most other retinal lesions, they tend to produce relative scotomata with indiscrete borders. Their location may be peripheral with central extension, or localized as with exudative detachment over a tumor or leaky blood vessels.

Ophthalmoscopy may sometimes confuse retinoschisis and retinal detachment, but a differentiation may be easily made by visual field examination. Visual field defects in retinoschisis tend to be quite deep with relatively sharp margins, having a characteristic peripheral location and dome shape extending centrally. These scotomata may be totally outside the central 30 degrees of field, and so a peripheral field test often must be used to detect them (figure 66). Visual field testing is also a good way to follow the central progression of retinoschisis.

It is possible occasionally to find field defects in glaucoma patients which are not caused by glaucoma and which can mislead the doctor about the extent and progress of the disease. Retinochoroiditis scars, for example, may produce field defects similar to those seen in glaucoma (figure 67).

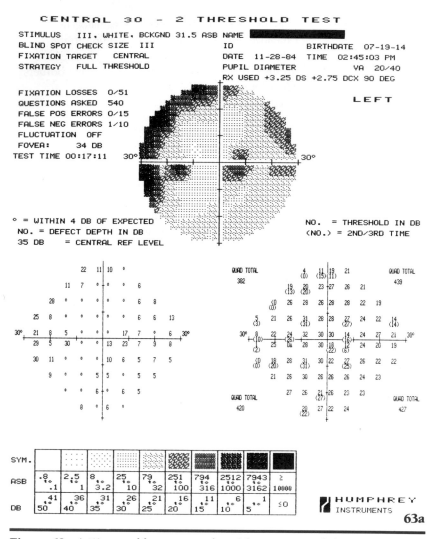

**Figure 63.** A 70-year-old man was referred for suspicion of glaucoma due to narrow angles and elevated tensions. Visual acuity was 20/20 OD and 20/40 OS. Intraocular pressure was 16 in each eye. The angles were narrow but not occludable. The cup/disc ratio was 0.25 in each eye.

A 30-2 threshold test revealed relative scotomata nasal to fixation in each eye with a tendency to break through to the superior field in each eye. (The superior temporal field defect found OS is a trial lens artifact.) Ophthalmoscopy disclosed irregular pigment epithelial changes, including "bone spicules" temporal to the macula OD and similar pigment changes OS.

A fluorescein angiogram showed pigment epithelial window defects around each macula and gutters directed inferiorly. The findings were consistent with old severe central serous chorioretinopathy. A repeat visual field six months later showed little change.

# CENTRAL 30 - 2 THRESHOLD TEST

STIMULUS   III, WHITE, BCKGND 31.5 ASB NAME ███████████
BLIND SPOT CHECK SIZE  III                ID                    BIRTHDATE  07-19-14
FIXATION TARGET   CENTRAL                 DATE  11-28-84  TIME  02:22:34 PM
STRATEGY   FULL THRESHOLD                 PUPIL DIAMETER                VA  20/20
                                          RX USED +3.25 DS +2.75 DCX 90 DEG

RIGHT

FIXATION LOSSES  1/46
QUESTIONS ASKED   479
FALSE POS ERRORS 0/17
FALSE NEG ERRORS 0/17
FLUCTUATION  OFF
          FOVEA:      36 DB
TEST TIME 00:14:53

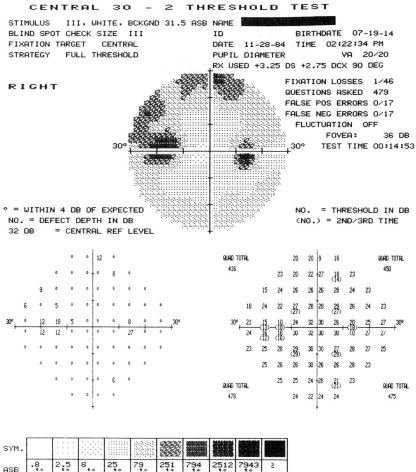

° = WITHIN 4 DB OF EXPECTED
NO. = DEFECT DEPTH IN DB
32 DB    = CENTRAL REF LEVEL

NO.  = THRESHOLD IN DB
(NO.) = 2ND/3RD TIME

```
            o   o | 12   o
         o    o   o|o   8   o
      9    o   5   o|o   o   o   o
   6    o   5   o|o   o   o   o   o
30°  o  |2 18  5  o|o   o   8   o   o  30°
     o  |2  12   o|o   o   o  27   o   o
      o    o   o   o|o   o   o   o   o
      o    o   o|o   o   o   o   o
         o    o   o|o   6   o
            o   o |o   o
```

```
QUAD TOTAL              20   20 |9    18        QUAD TOTAL
  416               23   20   22 +27   18   23      450
                                       (14)
              15   24   26   26 |26   28   24   23
         18   24   22   27   28 |28   29   26   24   23
                        (27)           (27)
30°  21   15   10   24   32 |30   26   20   25   27   30°
     24   (13) (10) 32   32 |30   30   (0)  27   27
          (18) (16)
          23   25   28   28  30 |30   27   28   27   25
                        (29)           (29)
               25   26   26   30 |26   26   28   23
QUAD TOTAL         25   25   24 +28   21   23    QUAD TOTAL
  478                              (21)              475
                   24   22 |24   24
```

| SYM. | | | | | | | | | | |
|---|---|---|---|---|---|---|---|---|---|---|
| ASB | .8 to .1 | 2.5 to 1 | 8 to 3.2 | 25 to 10 | 79 to 32 | 251 to 100 | 794 to 316 | 2512 to 1000 | 7943 to 3162 | ≥ 10000 |
| DB | 41 to 50 | 36 to 40 | 31 to 35 | 26 to 30 | 21 to 25 | 16 to 20 | 11 to 15 | 6 to 10 | 1 to 5 | ≤0 |

**HUMPHREY INSTRUMENTS**

**63b**

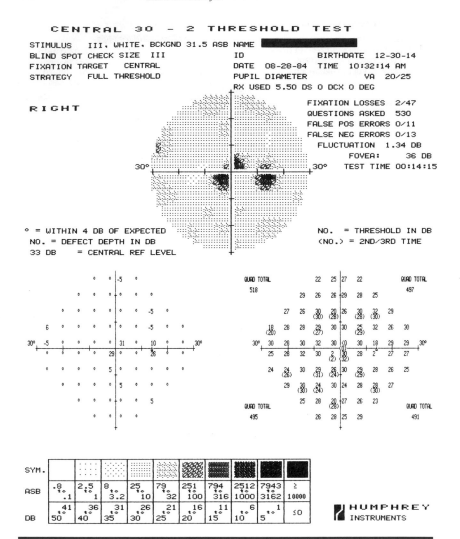

**Figure 64.** A 69-year-old woman volunteered to be a subject in a clinical evaluation of the Humphrey Field Analyzer. General medical and eye histories were unremarkable. Perimetric testing with the 30-2 threshold test revealed two deep and consistent scotomata near the fovea, one supra-temporal, and the other infero-nasal, about 4 degrees from fixation. The defects did not extend to the fovea; her foveal threshold was normal, and corrected acuity was 20/25. Fluorescein angiography displayed multiple window defects, which correlated in location with the para-central scotomata. The diagnosis was involutional macular degeneration.

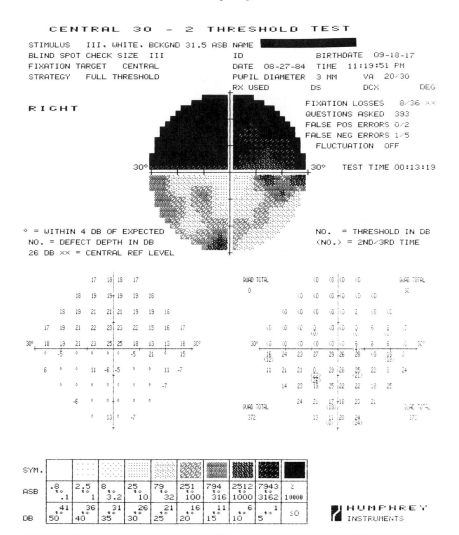

**Figure 65.** A 66-year-old man with a history of retinal artery obstruction in the left eye in 1982 came in for examination in 1984, reporting acute visual loss in the right eye. His vision at that time was finger counting. Fundus examination in the right eye revealed a refractive plaque in the central retinal artery just prior to branching on the disc. There was diffuse retinal edema over the posterior pole and a narrowing arterial blood column.

The patient was treated with massage, retrobulbar anesthesia, and paracentesis. His post-treatment accuity was 20/30 with a dense superior altitudinal field defect. This patient exhibits a branch retinal artery occlusion with inferior hemiretinal infarcation.

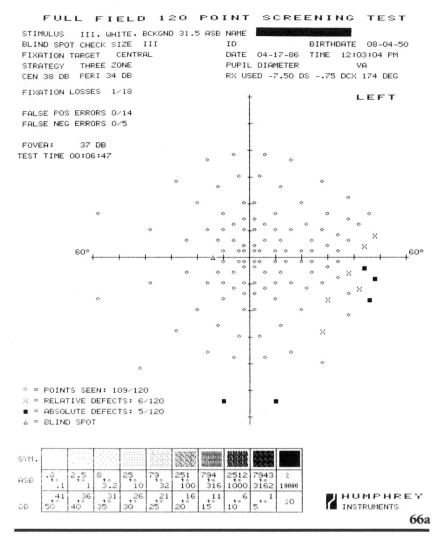

| SYM. |  |  |  |  |  |  |  |  |  |  |
|---|---|---|---|---|---|---|---|---|---|---|
| ASB | .8 to .1 | 2.5 to 1 | 8 to 3.2 | 25 to 10 | 79 to 32 | 251 to 100 | 794 to 316 | 2512 to 1000 | 7943 to 3162 | ≥ 10000 |
| DB | 41 to 50 | 36 to 40 | 31 to 35 | 26 to 30 | 21 to 25 | 16 to 20 | 11 to 15 | 6 to 10 | 1 to 5 | ≤0 |

HUMPHREY INSTRUMENTS

**66a**

**Figure 66.** A highly myopic 35-year-old woman presented for examination complaining of a foreign body sensation and general ache in the right eye. Slit lamp biomicroscopy showed quiet anterior segments in both eyes. Fundus examination revealed bilateral temporal retinoschisis extending to within approximately six disk diameters of the fovea OD, and eight disk diameters OS. Multiple inner wall holes were noted OU.

Perimetric screening using the 120-point full field test showed dense losses in the peripheral nasal fields OU, extending inward to within 40 degrees from fixation OS (figure 66a), and to within 30 degrees OD (figure 66b). Peripheral threshold testing with the Field Analyzer 30/60-2 threshold test confirmed these findings (figures 66c and 66d) and further quantified the extent of the field loss.

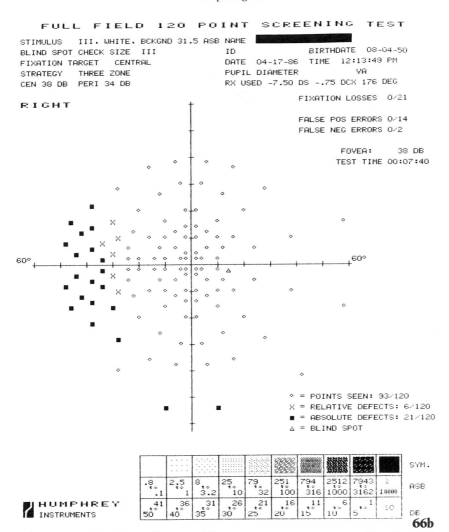

FULL FIELD 120 POINT SCREENING TEST

STIMULUS   III. WHITE, BCKGND 31.5 ASB   NAME ███████████
BLIND SPOT CHECK SIZE   III                      ID                    BIRTHDATE  08-04-50
FIXATION TARGET   CENTRAL                    DATE  04-17-86   TIME  12:13:49 PM
STRATEGY   THREE ZONE                          PUPIL DIAMETER              VA
CEN 38 DB  PERI 34 DB                            RX USED -7.50 DS -.75 DCX 176 DEG

FIXATION LOSSES  0/21

RIGHT

FALSE POS ERRORS 0/14
FALSE NEG ERRORS 0/2

FOVEA:      38 DB
TEST TIME 00:07:40

60°                                                              60°

○ = POINTS SEEN: 93/120
X = RELATIVE DEFECTS: 6/120
■ = ABSOLUTE DEFECTS: 21/120
△ = BLIND SPOT

| SYM. | | | | | | | | | | |
|------|--|--|--|--|--|--|--|--|--|--|
| ASB | .8 to .1 | 2.5 to 1 | 8 to 3.2 | 25 to 10 | 79 to 32 | 251 to 100 | 794 to 316 | 2512 to 1000 | 7943 to 3162 | ≥ 10000 |
| DB | 41 to 50 | 36 to 40 | 31 to 35 | 26 to 30 | 21 to 25 | 16 to 20 | 11 to 15 | 6 to 10 | 1 to 5 | ≤0 |

HUMPHREY
INSTRUMENTS

**66b**

PERIPH 30/60 - 2 THRESHOLD TEST

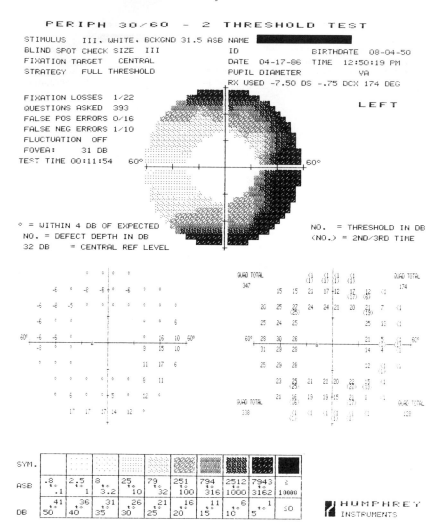

STIMULUS    III, WHITE, BCKGND 31.5 ASB  NAME ▮▮▮▮▮▮▮▮▮▮
BLIND SPOT CHECK SIZE  III              ID              BIRTHDATE  08-04-50
FIXATION TARGET   CENTRAL               DATE  04-17-86  TIME  12:50:19 PM
STRATEGY   FULL THRESHOLD               PUPIL DIAMETER          VA
                                        RX USED -7.50 DS -.75 DCX 174 DEG

FIXATION LOSSES  1/22
QUESTIONS ASKED   393                                           LEFT
FALSE POS ERRORS 0/16
FALSE NEG ERRORS 1/10
FLUCTUATION  OFF
FOVEA:      31 DB
TEST TIME 00:11:54      60°                          60°

° = WITHIN 4 DB OF EXPECTED                NO.  = THRESHOLD IN DB
NO. = DEFECT DEPTH IN DB                   <NO.> = 2ND/3RD TIME
32 DB   = CENTRAL REF LEVEL

| SYM. | | | | | | | | | | |
|---|---|---|---|---|---|---|---|---|---|---|
| ASB | .8 to .1 | 2.5 to 1 | 8 to 3.2 | 25 to 10 | 79 to 32 | 251 to 100 | 794 to 316 | 2512 to 1000 | 7943 to 3162 | ≥ 10000 |
| DB | 41 to 50 | 36 to 40 | 31 to 35 | 26 to 30 | 21 to 25 | 16 to 20 | 11 to 15 | 6 to 10 | 1 to 5 | ≤0 |

◪ HUMPHREY
  INSTRUMENTS

**66c**

PERIPH 30/60 - 2 THRESHOLD TEST

STIMULUS  III, WHITE, BCKGND 31.5 ASB NAME ████████
BLIND SPOT CHECK SIZE  III          ID                    BIRTHDATE  08-04-50
FIXATION TARGET  CENTRAL            DATE  04-17-86  TIME  12:34:18 PM
STRATEGY  FULL THRESHOLD            PUPIL DIAMETER            VA
                                    RX USED -7.50 DS -.75 DCX 176 DEG

RIGHT                               FIXATION LOSSES  0/24
                                    QUESTIONS ASKED  432
                                    FALSE POS ERRORS 0/18
                                    FALSE NEG ERRORS 0/9
                                    FLUCTUATION  OFF
                                        FOVEA:    29 DB
           60°            60°        TEST TIME 00:12:44

° = WITHIN 4 DB OF EXPECTED              NO.  = THRESHOLD IN DB
NO. = DEFECT DEPTH IN DB                 <NO.> = 2ND/3RD TIME
33 DB  = CENTRAL REF LEVEL

| SYM. | | | | | | | | | | |
|---|---|---|---|---|---|---|---|---|---|---|
| ASB | .8 to .1 | 2.5 to 1 | 8 to 3.2 | 25 to 10 | 79 to 32 | 251 to 100 | 794 to 316 | 2512 to 1000 | 7943 to 3162 | 2 10000 |
| DB | 41 to 50 | 36 to 40 | 31 to 35 | 26 to 30 | 21 to 25 | 16 to 20 | 11 to 15 | 6 to 10 | 1 to 5 | ≤0 |

HUMPHREY INSTRUMENTS

**66d**

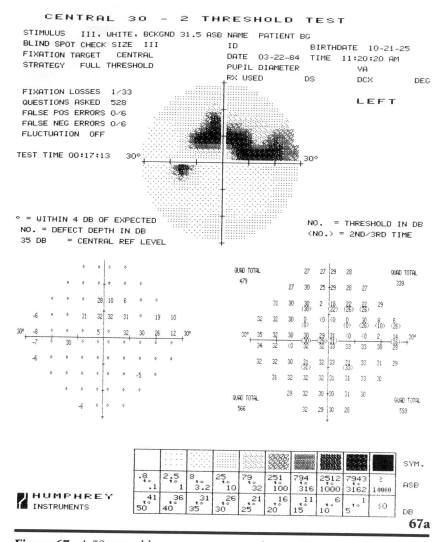

**Figure 67.** A 58-year-old woman was seen with complaints relating to her spectacle correction. Both general medical and ophthalmological histories were unremarkable. Routine dilated fundus examination showed an old, punched out retinal lesion about one disk diameter in size, immediately infero-temporal to the disk. Threshold perimetric testing showed a corresponding arcuate field defect similar to that which might be expected in glaucoma. All other eye findings were within normal limits.

Juxtapapillary choroiditis can produce field defects which may be incorrectly ascribed to glaucoma. Careful ophthalmoscopic evaluation of the posterior pole is required, as such lesions may be quite small.

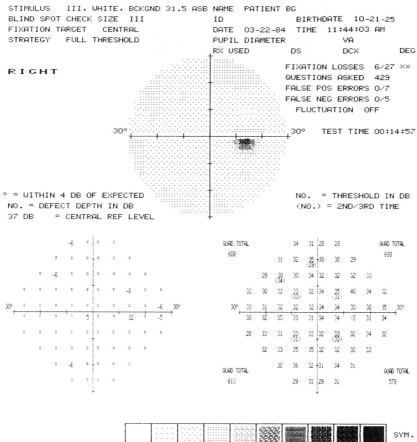

CENTRAL 30 - 2 THRESHOLD TEST

STIMULUS    III, WHITE, BCKGND 31.5 ASB  NAME   PATIENT BG
BLIND SPOT CHECK SIZE   III          ID              BIRTHDATE  10-21-25
FIXATION TARGET   CENTRAL            DATE  03-22-84  TIME  11:44:03 AM
STRATEGY   FULL THRESHOLD            PUPIL DIAMETER          VA
                                     RX USED        DS      DCX        DEG

RIGHT

FIXATION LOSSES   6/27 ××
QUESTIONS ASKED   429
FALSE POS ERRORS 0/7
FALSE NEG ERRORS 0/5
FLUCTUATION   OFF

30°                              30°    TEST TIME 00:14:57

° = WITHIN 4 DB OF EXPECTED                  NO.  = THRESHOLD IN DB
NO. = DEFECT DEPTH IN DB                    (NO.) = 2ND/3RD TIME
37 DB    = CENTRAL REF LEVEL

HUMPHREY
INSTRUMENTS

67b

# ARTIFACTS: FALSE FIELD DEFECTS

O NE COMMON error in interpreting test results can arise when the practitioner overlooks the effects of ordinary physical factors on test results and interprets them as field defects. Figure 68 shows a large number of combined threshold fields of normal right eyes with the peripheral and central fields merged. Notice that it is normal for facial anatomy and eyelids to produce significant restrictions in the superior, nasal and inferior fields.

One major source of false "field defects" in test results is physiological ptosis, or droopy lid, which can appear on the test results as a total or relative lack of sensitivity in the upper area of the field (figure 69). This particular problem is more common in computerized perimetry than it is in manual perimetry, probably because while manual perimetry tends to work in a single area of the field at a time, computerized perimetry uses a random stimulus sequence so the patient cannot anticipate where the next stimulus will come from. This improves fixation, but it decreases the incentive for the patient to keep his or her eyes more open than he normally would.

Another type of false field defect is caused by angioscotomata, or microscotomata which are not picked up by kinetic perimetry. In static perimetry, however, a stimulus may occasionally flash in just the place where the blood vessel is enlarged and the patient doesn't see. These defects commonly occur around the blind spot.

A similar source of false field defects that should be considered are refractive scotomata caused by small variations in retinal topography. In this situation, one portion of the retina may be significantly myopic or hyperopic relative to another. Images which are focused well in one part of the field may be significantly blurred in another area, giving the impression of a field defect for refractive reasons alone. It is not uncommon, for example, for the optic discs to be tilted and to be thus associated with such a variation in retinal topography. When this condition occurs bilaterally, as it often does, the effect may be to mimic a bitemporal field loss. Before CT scans became common, patients with refractive scotomata were sometimes even referred for pituitary tumor surgery.

It is important to record pupil size at the time of testing because extreme variations in pupil size may affect test results and, in some cases, give a false impression of field loss (figure 70). An incorrect prescription or the lack of a trial lens when it is needed may also sometimes give the impression of field loss (figure 71).

A final type of false defect is caused by the rim of the trial lens and appears in the periphery of the central visual field. High plus correction limits the size of the field within the trial lens. A classic example, of course, is the limited field in corrected aphakia (figure 72). The lens rim can also cause test results that look like peripheral field defects if the patient moves and gets misaligned from the corrective lens (figure 73). One should interpret areas which look like field defects but which are visible only 25° or more out in the field with caution. One way to minimize this effect is to bring the trial lens as close to the patient's eye as possible.

Statpac analysis can usually eliminate test result interference caused by the most commonly seen brow and eyelid artifacts, but if trial lenses are improperly positioned, the interference with test results will also appear in the statistical analysis. When in doubt, retest without the trial lens.

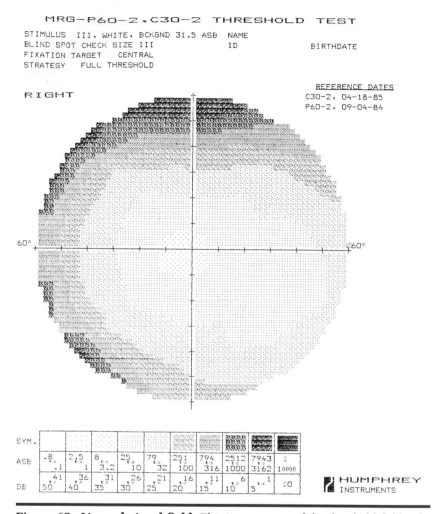

MRG-P60-2.C30-2 THRESHOLD TEST

STIMULUS III, WHITE, BCKGND 31.5 ASB   NAME
BLIND SPOT CHECK SIZE III              ID              BIRTHDATE
FIXATION TARGET   CENTRAL
STRATEGY   FULL THRESHOLD

REFERENCE DATES
C30-2, 04-18-85
P60-2, 09-04-84

RIGHT

60°     60°

**Figure 68. Normal visual field.** This is an average of the threshold fields of a large number of normal right eyes. Both central and peripheral results are shown merged together on one page. Notice that it is normal to have significant restrictions in the superior, nasal, and inferior fields, simply due to facial anatomy and eyelid effects. These factors are, of course, much less at issue when considering only the central field, but even there lid effects can be significant, especially in older patients.

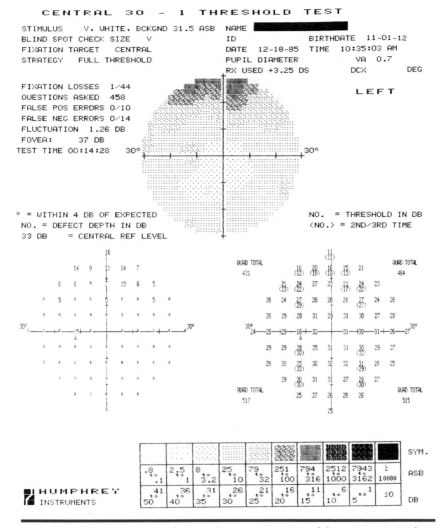

**Figure 69.** The apparent defects in the upper portion of this patient's visual field are caused by a drooping eyelid.

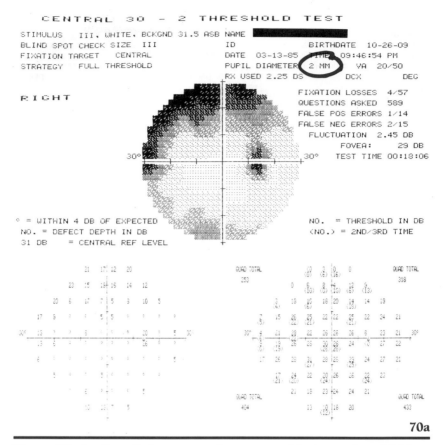

**70a**

**Figure 70.** Small pupil size can sometimes create a false impression of field defects on test results. When this 76-year-old patient was first tested, his pupil size was constricted to 2 mm and the test results indicated some field loss (figure 70a). The patient was tested later with the pupil dilated to 8 mm. Note that with dilation some field loss is still apparent, but that the overall sensitivity has increased significantly (figure 70b). It is important to record the patient's pupil size during testing as an aid to interpreting test results.

The 31.5 asb background illumination level used with the Humphrey and Goldmann perimeters was chosen to minimize the effects of variations in pupil size. Nevertheless, the extreme change from 2 mm to 8mm illustrated here was associated with an average increase in sensitivity of over 5 dB. A few decibels of this increase may well have been associated with learning effects or long-term fluctuations. The balance of the difference was likely to be due to the pilocarpine-induced miosis during the first test and the sixteen-fold increase in pupillary area in the second test. Perimeters operating at background levels lower than the 31.5 asb used by the Humphrey and Goldmann perimeters may be expected to be much more susceptible to this effect (Heuer, Gressel, Anderson et al. 1985; Klewin and Radius 1986).

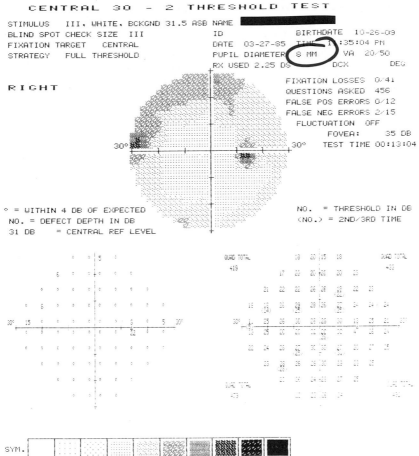

CENTRAL 30 - 2 THRESHOLD TEST

STIMULUS   III, WHITE, BCKGND 31.5 ASB NAME
BLIND SPOT CHECK SIZE   III                    ID                    BIRTHDATE  10-26-09
FIXATION TARGET    CENTRAL                      DATE  03-27-85   TIME   1:35:04 PM
STRATEGY   FULL THRESHOLD                       PUPIL DIAMETER  8 MM     VA   20/50
                                                RX USED 2.25 DS      DCX        DEG

RIGHT                                           FIXATION LOSSES   0/41
                                                QUESTIONS ASKED   456
                                                FALSE POS ERRORS 0/12
                                                FALSE NEG ERRORS 2/15
                                                FLUCTUATION  OFF
                                                       FOVEA:      35 DB
                    30°                   30°    TEST TIME 00:13:04

° = WITHIN 4 DB OF EXPECTED                     NO.  = THRESHOLD IN DB
NO. = DEFECT DEPTH IN DB                        (NO.) = 2ND/3RD TIME
31 DB    = CENTRAL REF LEVEL

| SYM. | | | | | | | | | |
|---|---|---|---|---|---|---|---|---|---|
| ASB | .8 to .1 | 2.5 to 1 | 8 to 3.2 | 25 to 10 | 79 to 32 | 251 to 100 | 794 to 316 | 2512 to 1000 | 7943 to 3162 | ≥ 10000 |
| DB | 41 to 50 | 36 to 40 | 31 to 35 | 26 to 30 | 21 to 25 | 16 to 20 | 11 to 15 | 6 to 10 | 1 to 5 | ≤0 |

HUMPHREY
INSTRUMENTS

**70b**

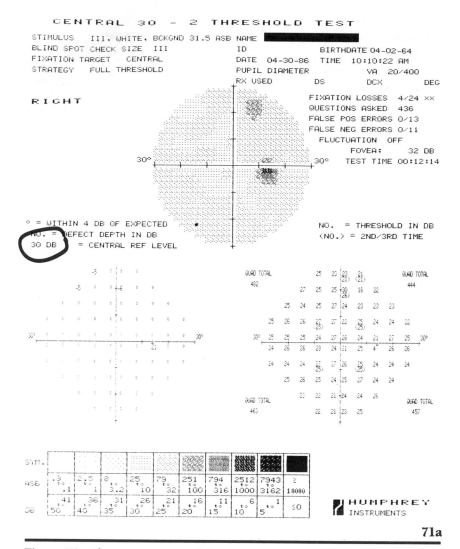

**Figure 71.** The apparent general depression in figure 71a was caused by a lack of refractive correction. When the test was run again with the proper trial lens in place (figure 71b), a much more representative measurement of the patient's visual field was obtained.

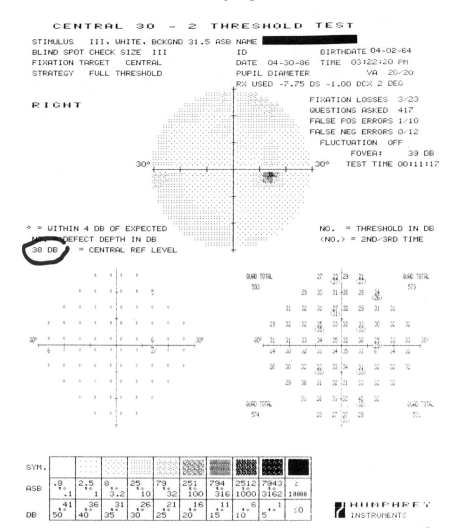

CENTRAL 30 - 2 THRESHOLD TEST

STIMULUS III, WHITE, BCKGND 31.5 ASB NAME ████████████████
BLIND SPOT CHECK SIZE III ID BIRTHDATE 04-02-64
FIXATION TARGET CENTRAL DATE 04-30-86 TIME 03:22:20 PM
STRATEGY FULL THRESHOLD PUPIL DIAMETER VA 20/20
RX USED -7.75 DS -1.00 DCX 2 DEG

RIGHT
FIXATION LOSSES 3/23
QUESTIONS ASKED 417
FALSE POS ERRORS 1/10
FALSE NEG ERRORS 0/12
FLUCTUATION OFF
FOVEA: 39 DB
30° 30° TEST TIME 00:11:17

° = WITHIN 4 DB OF EXPECTED NO. = THRESHOLD IN DB
NO. = DEFECT DEPTH IN DB (NO.) = 2ND/3RD TIME
38 DB = CENTRAL REF LEVEL

| SYM. | | | | | | | | | | |
|---|---|---|---|---|---|---|---|---|---|---|
| ASB | .8 to .1 | 2.5 to 1 | 8 to 3.2 | 25 to 10 | 79 to 32 | 251 to 100 | 794 to 316 | 2512 to 1000 | 7943 to 3162 | ≥ 10000 |
| DB | 41 to 50 | 36 to 40 | 31 to 35 | 26 to 30 | 21 to 25 | 16 to 20 | 11 to 15 | 6 to 10 | 1 to 5 | ≤0 |

HUMPHREY
INSTRUMENTS

71b

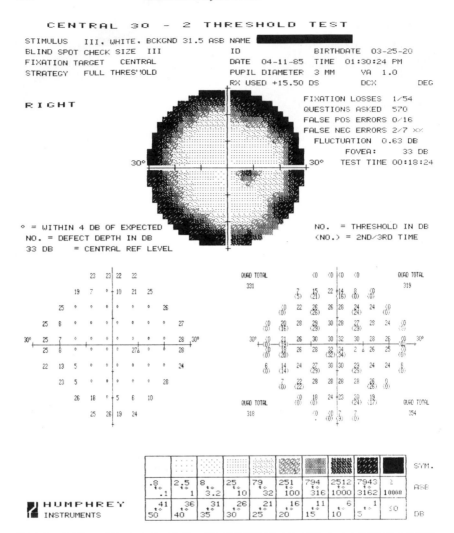

**Figure 72.** The apparent defects ringing this aphakic patient's central visual field are caused by the rim of the trial lens. False defects of this type are not eliminated by Statpac analysis.

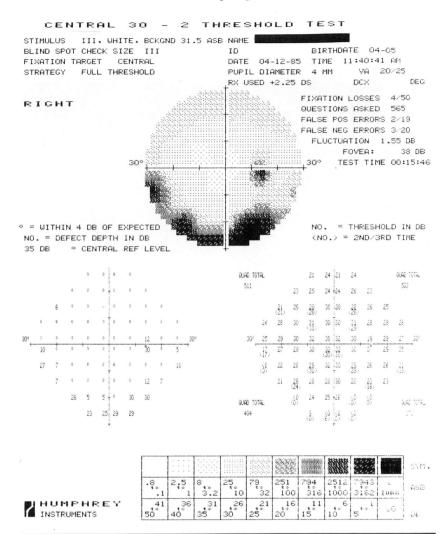

**Figure 73.** The defect in the lower portion of the visual field is caused by the misaligned rim of the trial lens.

# 6.

# Interpreting Test Results With Statpac

THE HUMPHREY FIELD ANALYZER'S statistical package, Statpac, can be used to produce an in-depth statistical analysis of visual field test results. Statpac performs three important functions: (1) it can point out suspicious areas that otherwise might not be evident until subsequent testing; (2) it can identify areas that look suspicious but which, in fact, compare favorably with normals data; and (3) using results from a series of tests, Statpac can provide a highly sensitive and informative analysis of changes in the patient's visual field over time.

The statistical package is based on an entirely new model of the visual field developed through extensive testing of normal visual fields. It compares test results with the model to determine how frequently the threshold result found at a given location in a patient's field occurs in the normal population. In addition to this point-by-point analysis, Statpac uses four global indices to indicate how much the height and shape of the patient's hill of vision deviate from the norm. All of these calculations are automatically corrected for the patient's age, year by year.

The statistical analyses can be printed in three formats: single field analysis, overview, and change analysis. The single field analysis, as its name implies, analyzes the results of a single threshold test. The overview presents the results of up to ten tests in four formats on one page for convenient comparison. The change analysis compares a series of tests and analyzes indices of change in the patient's field over time, flagging significant indicators for the doctor's attention. (Detailed instructions for performing Statpac analyses can be found in the *Statpac User's Guide*).

# THE SINGLE FIELD ANALYSIS PRINTOUT

**S**TATPAC'S SINGLE FIELD ANALYSIS (figure 74) shows the result of a single central threshold test. The top of the page presents patient data, test reliability indices, and test results in the grayscale and numeric formats standard for Field Analyzer threshold test results. The information that Statpac adds is found in the lower half of the page.

## Total Deviation Plots

On the left in the lower half of the single field analysis printout is a pair of plots, one above the other, labeled "total deviation." The numeric values in the upper plot represent the difference in decibels between the patient's test results and the age-corrected normal values at each tested point in the visual field.

The lower total deviation plot, called a probability plot, translates the values in the upper plot into grayscale symbols. These are explained in the little chart labeled "probability symbols" to the right of the total deviation probability plot. The darker the symbol the less likely it is that the field is normal in that location. For instance, a totally black square indicates that the deviation from normal found at that point location occurs in less than 0.5% of normal subjects; such a point must then be regarded as highly suspect. Notice that this probability statement is made on a point-by-point basis, allowing the practitioner to read results like an isopter plot or grayscale.

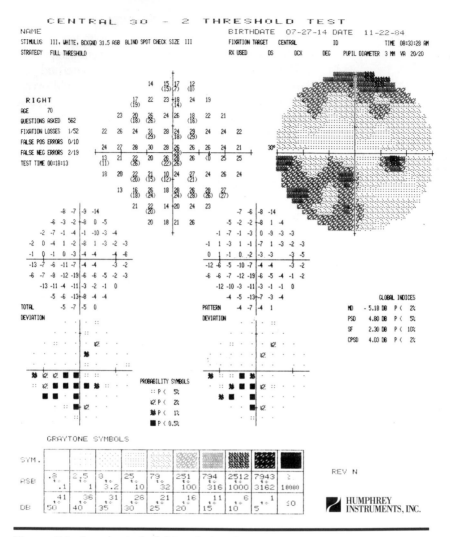

**Figure 74.** Sample single field analysis printout

## Pattern Deviation Plots

Further to the right in the single field analysis printout are two more plots, one above the other, labeled "pattern deviation." These are similar to the total deviation plots, except that here Statpac has adjusted the analysis of the test results for any overall changes in the height of the measured hill of vision caused, for example, by such things as cataracts or small pupils. Similarly, Statpac also corrects for any patients who are "supernormal," adjusting the expected hill of vision upward by the appropriate amount and thereby making the analysis more sensitive to localized scotomata.

Thus, the numeric pattern deviation plot shows the deviation in decibels from the age-corrected normal values, adjusted for any shift in overall sensitivity. The probability pattern deviation plot indicates the statistical significance of the result at each point. Again, the darker the symbol the more significant the deviation from the expected threshold.

For a comparison of the differences in the information provided by the total deviation and pattern deviation plots look ahead to figure 80b. Note that as the patient's cataract causes an increasing overall field loss, both the grayscale and the probability symbols in the total deviation plots grow darker. The total deviation plot is indicating the degree to which the patient's field deviates from age normals. The probability symbols in the pattern deviation plot, on the other hand, do not gradually darken. That is because pattern deviation corrects for any depression in the overall field, making it possible to track localized scotomata in the presence of a media opacity.

## Foveal Threshold

If the foveal threshold option was chosen when the test was run, the Field Analyzer will print the measured value just below the test time on the upper left side of the page. When the patient's foveal threshold is significantly depressed, a probability symbol will appear next to the value shown. This symbol is identical to those used for the probability plots and indicates the significance of the deviation from age normal.

# Global Indices

Finally, a short chart labeled "global indices" appears on the far right side of the page. Here Statpac has made some calculations to provide overall guidelines to help the practitioner assess the field results as a whole rather than on the point-by-point basis shown in the total deviation and pattern deviation plots. Because the four global indices are calculated from deviations from age-corrected normals data, the p values for the global indices, discussed below, are not corrected again for age. The four global indices are mean deviation (MD), pattern standard deviation (PSD), short-term fluctuation (SF), and corrected pattern standard deviation (CPSD).

**MD**  MD is the mean elevation or depression of the patient's overall field compared to the normal reference field. In figure 74, for example, on the average, this patient's tests results were 5.18 dB below the norm. If the deviation is significantly outside the population norms, a p value is given, in this case 2%. This means that less than 2% of the normal population shows an MD larger than the value found in this test. Categories for p values are $p < 10\%$, $p < 5\%$, $p < 2\%$, $p < 1\%$ and $p < 0.5\%$.

A significant MD may indicate that the patient has an overall depression, or that there is loss in one part of the field and not in others. MD is best interpreted in relation to the total and pattern deviation charts.

**PSD**  PSD stands for pattern standard deviation. PSD is a measurement of the degree to which the shape of the patient's measured field departs from the normal, age-corrected reference field. A low PSD indicates a smooth hill of vision. A high PSD indicates an irregular hill and may be due either to variability in patient response or to actual field irregularities.

To indicate the statistical significance of the calculated PSD the Field Analyzer uses the same categories for p as with the mean deviation. In figure 74 the patient's PSD is 4.81 dB, and the p value is $<5\%$. This means that less than 5% of the normal population shows a PSD larger than the value found in this test.

**SF**  SF is short-term fluctuation, which the Field
Analyzer has been measuring all along. It is an index
of the consistency of the patient's answers during
the test and is obtained by testing twice at ten pre-
selected points. The SF found for the patient in figure
74 is 2.32 dB, and the p value is <10%. This
means that less than 10% of the normal population
shows an SF value larger than the value found in
this test. Categories for p value are the same as for MD.

When a test is run using Field Analyzer software
that includes Statpac, the fluctuation test is turned on
automatically. It can be turned off, but because this
measurement is used in calculating CPSD (see below),
it is best to leave it on.

**CPSD**  CPSD stands for corrected pattern standard
deviation. It is a measure of how much the total shape
of the patient's hill of vision deviates from the shape
of the hill of vision normal for the patient's age,
after correcting for intra-test variability. The hill of
vision may be irregular in shape because of unreliable
patient response, because of actual field losses, or a
combination of the two factors. The CPSD in figure 74,
for example, is 4.04 dB and the p value is <2%.
This means that less than 2% of the normal population
shows a CPSD value larger than the value found in
the this test. Categories for p values are the same as for
MD.

In calculating CPSD, Statpac attempts to remove the
effects of patient variability during the test and to
present only the irregularity caused by actual field loss.
CPSD depends on both PSD and SF and is therefore
not available unless the fluctuation option was turned
on during the test.

Figure 75 shows the single field analysis of threshold
test results which were presented earlier in figure
49. Statpac can, of course, be used with stored test
results. The practitioner chose not to use the fluctuation
option when the tests were originally done, and
while the analysis is still quite informative, note that
the word "off" appears next to the SF and CPSD
instead of a calculated value.

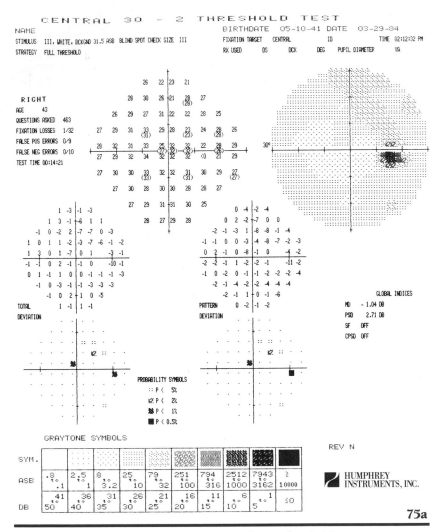

**Figure 75.** Humphrey Field Analyzer central 30-2 threshold tests were run nine months apart on the right eye of a 43-year-old man with pigmentary glaucoma. The case description and original test results for this patient are shown in figure 49 on page 74. The Statpac single field analysis of those test results is shown here.

In the single field analysis of the first test (figure 75a) both the total and pattern deviation plots show a pattern of significant loss in the superior temporal arcuate area, plus a single point just supero-nasal to fixation, none of which are strongly highlighted by the conventional grayscale. Neither the mean

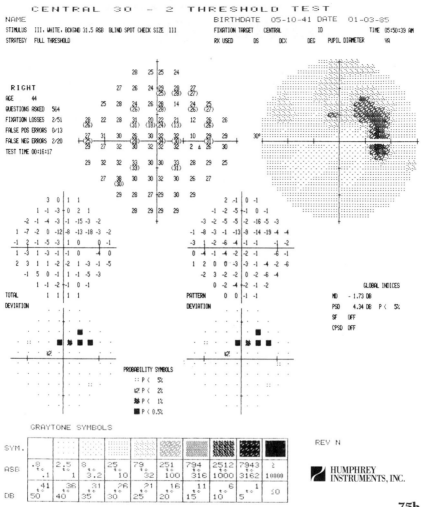

CENTRAL 30 - 2 THRESHOLD TEST

NAME                                  BIRTHDATE  05-10-41  DATE  01-03-85

STIMULUS  III, WHITE, BCKGND 31.5 ASB  BLIND SPOT CHECK SIZE  III      FIXATION TARGET  CENTRAL     ID     TIME 05:50:39 AM

STRATEGY  FULL THRESHOLD                       RX USED   DS   DCX   DEG   PUPIL DIAMETER   VA

RIGHT
AGE  44
QUESTIONS ASKED  564
FIXATION LOSSES  2/51
FALSE POS ERRORS  0/13
FALSE NEG ERRORS  2/20
TEST TIME 00:16:17

GLOBAL INDICES

MD  - 1.73 DB
PSD  4.34 DB  P < 5%
SF  OFF
CPSD  OFF

PROBABILITY SYMBOLS

:: P < 5%
▨ P < 2%
▩ P < 1%
■ P < 0.5%

GRAYTONE SYMBOLS

| SYM. | | | | | | | | | |
|---|---|---|---|---|---|---|---|---|---|
| ASB | .8 to .1 | 2.5 to 1 | 8 to 3.2 | 25 to 10 | 79 to 32 | 251 to 100 | 794 to 316 | 2512 to 1000 | 7943 to 3162 | ≥ 10000 |
| DB | 41 to 50 | 36 to 40 | 31 to 35 | 26 to 30 | 21 to 25 | 16 to 20 | 11 to 15 | 6 to 10 | 1 to 5 | ≤0 |

REV N

 HUMPHREY INSTRUMENTS, INC.

**75b**

deviation nor the PSD global indices depart significantly from the population norms. Statpac analysis of follow-up test results (figure 75b) showed further development of field loss in these areas; by this time the defect was apparent on the conventional grayscale.

# THE OVERVIEW PRINTOUT

**S**TATPAC'S OVERVIEW PRINTOUT (figure 76) can show the results of up to ten tests on one page. This presentation of test results makes it easier to review the results of a series of tests without having to clear a large table to lay them all out. The tests are automatically printed in chronological order. The patient's name, birthdate, the type of test, and eye tested appear at the top of the page.

The overview printout presents the results of each test in four formats: standard grayscale, standard dB numeric, a total deviation probability plot, and a pattern deviation probability plot. The date of each test appears to the upper left of the grayscale presentation, and the visual acuity and pupil size are printed to the upper right of the pattern deviation probability plot. The fixation losses, false negative and false positive scores appear just above the four test result presentations. Below the test results are printed the foveal threshold and the same four global indices used in the single analysis. The key to the probability symbols appears in the lower right corner of the page.

Figure 80b offers a good example of the summary value of the overview format. Although the small pages of this *Primer* do not allow the presentation of a full printout of ten test results, even with the five results that can be shown here the progress of the patient's cataract and the effect of surgery are readily apparent on a single page.

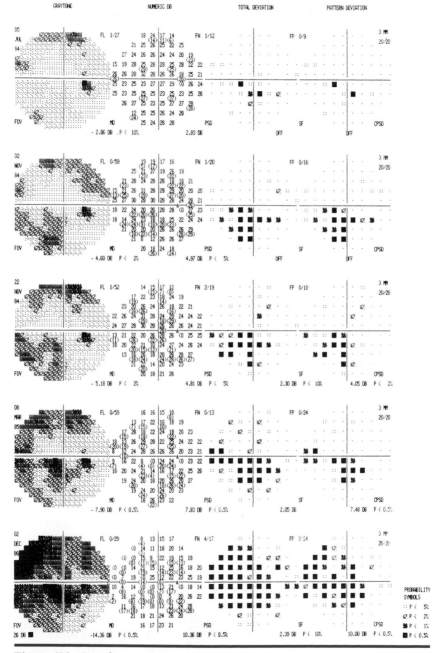

**Figure 76.** Sample overview printout

# THE CHANGE ANALYSIS PRINTOUT

L IKE THE OVERVIEW PRINTOUT, the change analysis printout (figure 77) shows the Statpac analyses of up to ten test results on one sheet. In this case, Statpac produces an analytical summary of changes in the patient's visual field from the time of the earliest test included in the summary to the time of the most recent test included.

Statpac presents the change analysis in the form of a box plot analysis of test results and a summary of four global indices. The indices are the same four presented in the single field analysis, but this time they are plotted over time to indicate changes in the patient's visual field.

## The Box Plot

Because the box plot, at first sight, is the hardest for non-statisticians to interpret, let's begin there. Box plots are helpful in making a quick determination about the nature and extent of visual field changes over time.

Look at the box plot in figure 78. The four main things to note are:

1. The overall shape of the box, how elongated or compact it is;
2. The location of the three dark lines inside the box that indicate the median (a);
3. The top and bottom end points of the line along which the box lies (b); and
4. Where the box is plotted against the normal scale on the left (see figure 77 for this).

For the statistically and mathematically-minded (everybody else just bear with us for a sentence or so), the box plot is a modified histogram that gives a five-number summary of the test results. The summary is made up of the differences at each tested point between the patient's measured field and Statpac's age-corrected reference field. Statpac plots the extreme values of these differences (the 100th and zero percentiles, or top and bottom end points of the line shown at (b) in figure 78), the median difference

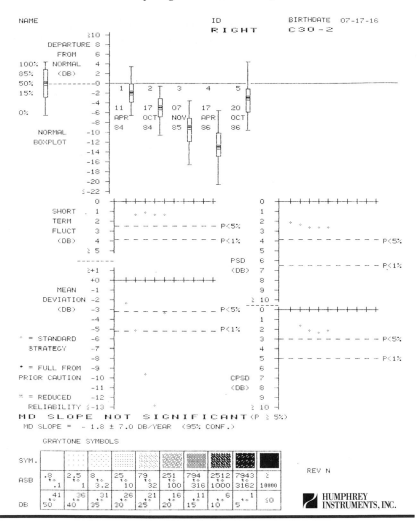

**Figure 77.** Sample change analysis printout

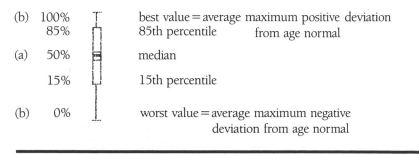

**Figure 78.** Normal box plot

(the three dark lines inside the box shown at (a) in figure 78), and the 85th and 15th percentile differences (the top and bottom of the box). To facilitate interpretation, a "normal" box is presented to the left of the scale. This is the average box drawn from the normals data on which the Statpac model is based.

The 100th percentile represents the patient's most sensitive tested point or points relative to age normals. In the test results for October 17, 1984, shown in figure 77, for example, the patient's most sensitive tested points were about 1 dB below the median results for age normals, or 5 dB below the best normal test results for people of the same age. Again, the 85th percentile for the same test falls at − 3 dB. This means that 85% of the patient's tested points differ from normal median values by − 3 dB or more, and from normal 85th percentile values by − 5 dB.

Because the patient in figure 77 (also shown as figure 79a) is suffering from cataract, the entire visual field is depressed more or less evenly, and the only change in the measured field is a general depression of sensitivity over time. Therefore, the shape of the box plot remains fairly normal, but the whole symbol is depressed.

This is not always the case. For example, a visual field with a deep scotoma covering a small number of points will result in a box plot in which the box is more or less normal in shape and location, and there is a long negative tail (figure 79b). When a scotoma deepens over time, the length of the tail increases. In the case shown in figure 79b, the patient's least sensitive tested points, indicated by the bottom of the tail at 0%, are at least 22 dB below the median values and 16 dB below the worst tested points for age normals. In fact, this patient's worst tested points are probably depressed below − 22 dB, or off the scale.

If the scotoma enlarges to involve more than 15% of the points tested, the lower limit of the box will be further depressed, and depending on the extent and gravity of the field loss, the box may be very elongated (figure 79c).

The box plot section of the change analysis printout gives the dates of the tests included in the analyses. The test pattern used for each is also indicated if you have chosen to present results from both central 24-2 and central 30-2 tests, or 24-1 and 30-1 tests.

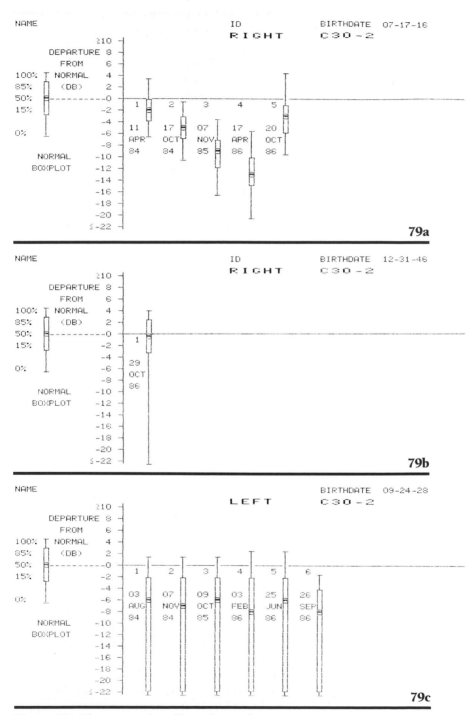

**Figure 79.** Three examples of box plot results

## Change Analysis Summary of Global Indices

The lower half of the change analysis printout displays summaries of the global indices MD (mean deviation), PSD (pattern standard deviation) SF (short-term fluctuation), and CPSD (corrected pattern standard deviation) for the tests shown in the box plot.

The summary results are presented chronologically and in the same order as in the box plots. Thus, test dates may be taken from the box plots.

To facilitate interpretation, the $p < 5\%$ and $p < 1\%$ limits for the normal population are shown as dashed reference lines. If, for example, the symbol indicating a test appears above the 5% line, the index value on the test is not significant at the 5% level. If it falls below the 5% line, the index value is significant at the 5% level. Similarly, if the symbol falls below the 1% line, the index value is significant at the 1% level; that is, less than 1% of the normal population shows an index value as large as or larger than that found in that test.

## Linear Regression Analysis

If five or more fields are analyzed on a change analysis printout, and all test results to be analyzed were run with the same strategy, Statpac will automatically perform a linear regression analysis of mean deviation (MD). One of two messages, "MD slope not significant" or "MD slope significant," will be printed below the MD plot when a linear regression analysis has been performed. The calculated slope in MD in decibels per year and the 95% confidence interval will also be printed.

A linear regression analysis tests the hypothesis that a slope is zero, that is, that there has been no change in the patient's visual field. If this hypothesis is rejected after analysis at the $p < 5\%$ level, the slope is said to be significant and the analysis continues at the 1% and 0.1% levels of significance. The result is then displayed as being significant at $p < 5\%$, $p < 1\%$, or $p < 0.1\%$.

It should be remembered that not only the significance level but also the magnitude of the slope is

important. In figure 80a, for example, the slope is
$-3.6$ dB per year, plus or minus 0.9. This means that
there is a 95% confidence level that the slope is
between $-2.7$ and $-4.5$ dB per year. The slope is
significant at the p level of less than 1%. This is
a slope magnitude on the order of more than thirty
times the rate of change due to aging in the normal
population. A slope of only one or two tenths of a
decibel per year would be viewed with considerably
less concern.

If the hypothesis that the slope is zero, that is, that
there has been no change in the patient's visual
field, is not rejected, the message "not significant"
appears and Statpac shows a p value of $\geq 5\%$,
indicating that the slope was not significant at the
largest p value Statpac is programmed to consider, 5%.

What does this mean clinically? a "significant"
message means that it is likely that mean deviation has
changed in the direction of the estimated slope, and
the lower the p value the more likely it is. However, it
remains for the clinician to establish whether this
indication on the test results is caused by progressive
field loss or by other factors.

The larger the number of tests analyzed, the more
easily small changes in MD are detected. A low
number of observations involves a higher risk that the
analysis will fail to detect a deterioration over time.

The application of the linear regression analysis
means that the following assumptions have been made:
1. The true MD changes linearly with time.
2. The differences between the measured and the
   true MD are independent, and identically
   and normally distributed.

## Messages and Cautions

As the explanatory chart on the lower left side of
the change analysis printout indicates, tests taken using
the standard full threshold strategy are identified
with (∴) and those using the full from prior data strategy
with (✳). The validity of applying Statpac analysis to
test results obtained with the full from prior strategy is
still under study as of this writing, and therefore a
caution notice appears when test results obtained with

that strategy are analyzed. Results from tests with poor reliability indices (high fixation losses, false positive, and false negative errors) are indicated by an X.

# COMBINING STATPAC ANALYSES

**T**HE USEFULNESS of performing more than one of the three available statistical analyses on a series of test results should be evident. Figure 80b has already been mentioned as a good example of the different kinds of information available from the total deviation and pattern deviation plots. This would be clear from one single field analysis of the third or fourth test results, but the overview gives additional quick summary of the progress of the patient's condition. The change analysis of the same five test results, shown in figure 80a, gives the practitioner further information about the significance of the changes seen in the test results over time.

Multiple statistical analyses were also performed for the patients whose test results are shown in figure 81, 82, and 83.

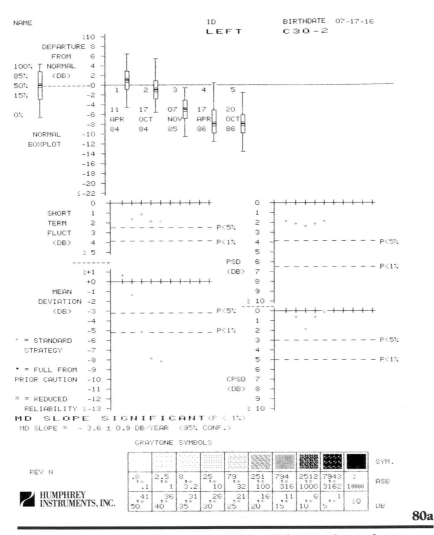

80a

**Figure 80.** A 70-year-old man had been followed for several years for management of elevated pressures OU, in the absence of field loss. Pressures had been 28 mm Hg OD, and 26 mm Hg OS prior to medication, and 20 OD and 17 OS after prescription of pilocarpine. Over a period of two years, starting in 1984, progressive field losses were seen in both eyes.

Look at the change analysis for the left eye (figure 80a). The mean deviation shows changes over time which are significant at the p <1% level; the MD slope is −3.6 dB per year. The box plots show the same significant drop in overall sensitivity, but note that the shape of the boxes closely resembles that of the normal boxplot. Also note that the plots of SF, PSD, and CPSD are all well within normal limits.

The picture here is one of overall depression of the hill of vision, with the

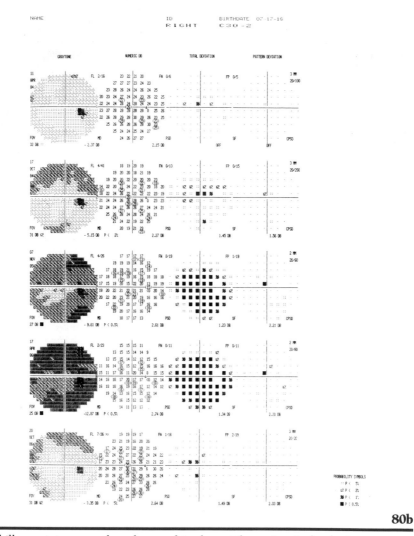

**80b**

hill remaining smooth and normal in shape. The patient is developing a cataract in this eye.

    The effects of the cataract on the right eye may also be seen on the overview printout (figure 80b). Scanning from the top to the bottom of the page, one can see that the grayscales gradually become darker, as do the total deviation plots. The pattern deviation plots, on the other hand, have remained normal during this same period. This illustrates the difference between total and pattern deviation. Total deviation shows departure from age normal values. Pattern deviation shows the same thing, but first corrects for any depression in the overall field, in this case a depression due to a cataract. The patient underwent cataract surgery between the fourth and fifth fields, and the results are clearly evident on the overview.

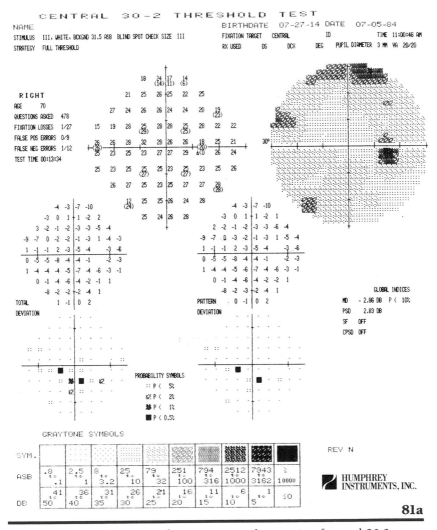

**Figure 81.** Over the course of seventeen months, a series of central 30-2 threshold tests was run on the right eye of a 70-year-old woman whose intraocular pressures had been known to be increased for at least ten years. The results of four Field Analyzer test taken during the first eight months and a case history are shown in figure 51 on page 78. A follow-up test and a Statpac analysis of all five test are shown here.

Look at the Statpac single field analysis of the first test, which was run in July of 1984 (figure 81a). The total and pattern deviation plots show significant deviations from normal at several points in the inferior field. These deviations are not readily apparent in the grayscale. The MD of − 2.86 dB shows that the average sensitivity is significantly reduced. This value is seen in less than 10% of the normal population (p <10%).

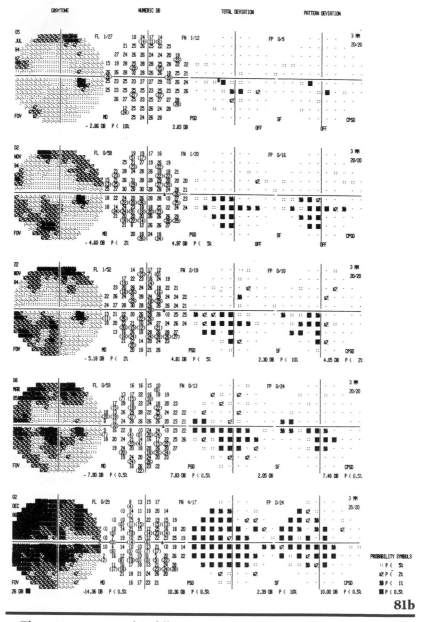

**81b**

The patient was tested in follow up and the results are shown in the overview printout (figure 81b) where definite and probably progressive defects are concentrated mainly in the inferior nasal visual field of the right eye.

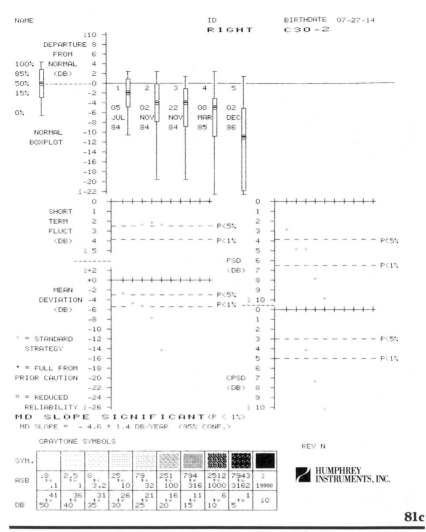

This progression is apparent in all four depictions of the test results in the overview format: the grayscale, numeric, total deviation, and pattern deviation plots.

Progression is also seen in the depiction of the global indices on the change analysis (figure 81c), where there are large changes in MD, PSD and CPSD. The change in MD was found to be significant at the p <0.1% level, with a slope of 4.6 ± 1.4 dB per year

A similar pattern may be seen in the box plots. Note that the descending tails on the box plots get longer with time, the boxes also elongate, and finally, the boxes move lower on the graph, all illustrating the general decay of the field.

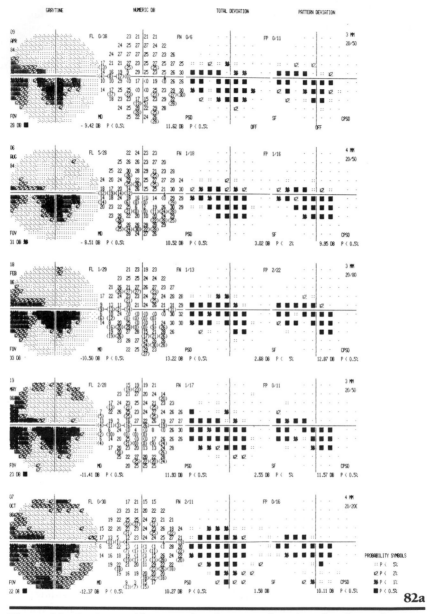

**Figure 82.** A 58-year-old man with a diagnosis of moderately advanced chronic open angle glaucoma underwent a laser trabeculoplasty in March of 1983. A series of fields taken in follow up are shown in the overview printout (figure 82a).

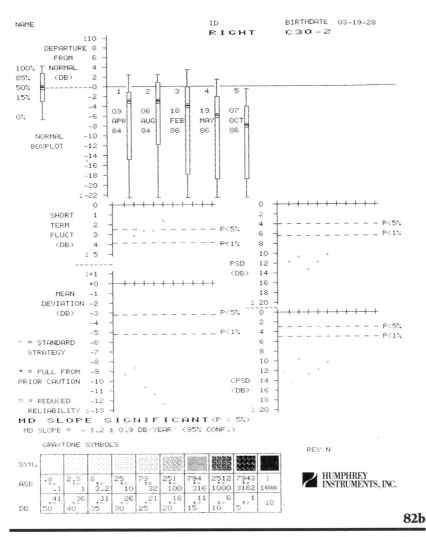

A change analysis performed after the fifth test confirms the impression of continued field loss (figure 82b). Note the position of the boxes, which are sinking on the scale but not elongating, suggesting that field loss is increasing overall. The global indices are well outside normal limits, and the MD shows a significant change at the p <5% level.

Such an overall increase in field loss may be caused by developing media opacity or by progression of the patient's glaucoma. The decrease in visual acuity from 20/50 to 20/200 suggests the former as the most likely diagnosis.

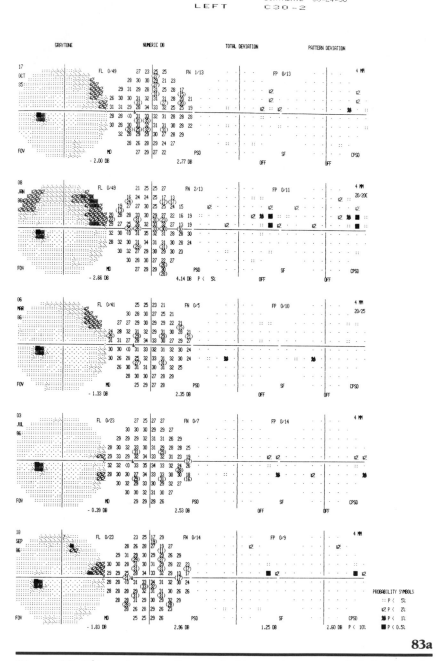

**Figure 83.** This patient was diagnosed with pseudotumor cerebri. A series of tests of the patient's right eye was performed over the course of a year, and the overview (figure 83a) shows the results of five of those tests. Look

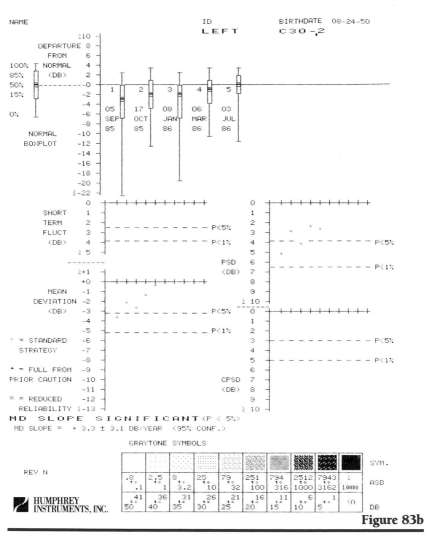

**Figure 83b**

at the change analysis performed after the July 1986 test (figure 83b). All indicators appear to show improvement in the visual field following the corrective surgery performed just prior to this test. The box plots are rising toward the normal level and becoming less elongated, and the descending tails are retracting. The MD also shows a generally upward trend, as reflected by the "MD slope significant" message with a p value of <5%. The slope was estimated at +3.3 dB per year.

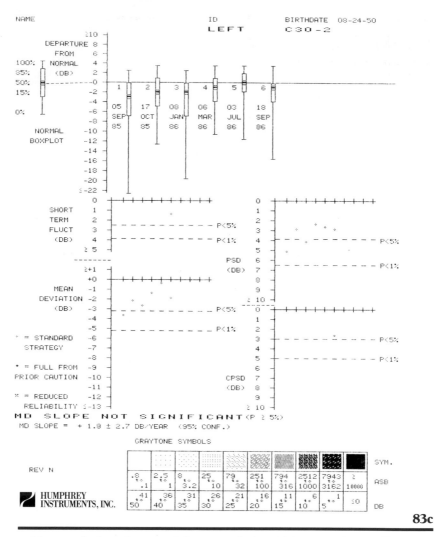

83c

However, look at the second change analysis, which covers six tests (figure 83c). The results of the sixth test are slightly worse than those of the fifth, and the MD slope is no longer significant. Slopes which are tagged as significant at p <5% may well be found to be marginally not significant upon subsequent testing. This is much less likely to happen when the p level is 1% or 0.1%, simply because 5% is the lowest level of significance classified in the linear regression analysis. For patients who show marginally significant field change, the value of repeated follow-up testing and further analysis of test results cannot be overstressed.

# STATPAC AND THE INDICES OF RELIABILITY

**A** S WE SAW in chapter 4, all Field Analyzer test result printouts show the number of fixation losses, and of false positive and false negative responses. These scores, known as reliability indices, help the practitioner determine the reliability of the patient's responses.

The visual fields used in developing Statpac were those of normal subjects whose reliability indices were within certain limits. Tests results showing fixation losses scores of 20% or more and false positive or false negative errors of 33% or more were excluded as unreliable. Therefore, if Statpac is used to analyze the test results of a patient whose reliability scores fall outside these limits, the analytical results must be regarded with caution.

The reliability indices appear on the single field analysis printout as they do on other Field Analyzer printouts and, as usual, the Field Analyzer prints an XX after scores that fall outside the established limits. In such cases, Statpac single field analysis printouts also include the message "low patient reliability makes comparison with normal data base questionable."

Look, for example, at the single field analysis printout shown in figure 84. This glaucoma patient came in for a follow-up test in July, 1986 and a Statpac analysis of the results was performed. Two notable aspects of the results and the analysis will be immediately apparent. First, note that Statpac has flagged the results in the upper left of the printout with the low patient reliability message. The high fixation losses and false positives score triggered this flag. Second, the grayscale presentation of test results shows several white patches in the central field. This was clearly a trigger happy patient who was pressing the response button repeatedly while the primary points were being tested rather than pressing the button in response to a seen stimulus. The white patches in the grayscale would appear in the non-Statpac printout as well.

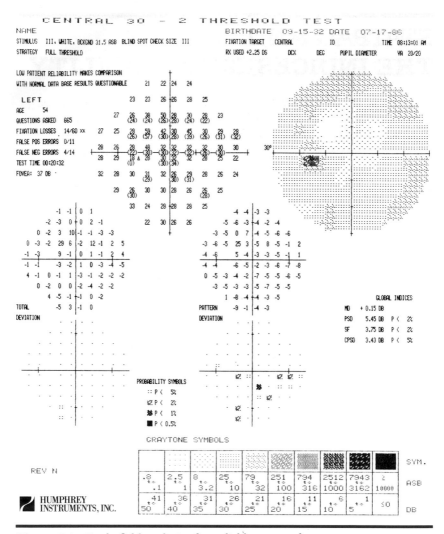

**Figure 84.** Single field analysis of unreliable test results

# A NOTE ON STATISTICS AND PROBABILITY

**W**HEN CONSIDERING the probability statements in this statistical package, it is important to be conscious of what they do and do not mean. They are an aid to interpretation, not a diagnosis. The doctor's judgement is still the most important element in determining the clinical significance of perimetric findings.

The probability statements are based on the distribution seen in the normal population. Saying that less than 5% of the normal population deviates from the norm by a certain amount means just that and no more. It does not mean that there is only a 5% chance that the result is normal.

The positive predictive rate depends, of course, on the prevalence of defective fields in the population studied. The probability that a given result is abnormal depends on the relative incidence in the population of defects caused by disease versus the incidence of the same field "defect" in normals. If a certain field result is seen 5% of the time in normals, and similar glaucomatous field defects are seen in 0.5% of the population, then the result is ten times as likely to be associated with normality as with disease.

Certainly one should also be aware that some patients commonly seen in a clinical practice may not meet the criteria of normality (for example, visual acuity) which had to be applied in creating a normals data base. These patients may fall outside normal limits established in this statistical package for reasons other than field loss, such as cataract.

# References Cited

Aulhorn, E. 1978. Visual field defects in chronic glaucoma. In *Glaucoma, Conceptions of a Disease: Pathogenesis, Diagnosis, Therapy,* ed. Heilman and Richardson, 157-168. Philadelphia: W.B. Saunders Company.

Aulhorn, E., and H. Harms. 1967. Early visual field defects in glaucoma. In *Glaucoma Symposium, Tutzing Castle,* 1966, ed. W. Leydhecker, 151-186. Basel, Switzerland: S. Karger.

———1972. Visual perimetry. *In Handbook of Sensory Physiology,* ed. Jameson and Hurvich, Vol. 7, No. 4, 102-145. Berlin: Springer-Verlag.

Bebie, H., F. Fankhauser, and J. Spahr. 1976. Static perimetry: accuracy and fluctuations. *Acta Opthal* 54:339-348.

Benedetto, M.D., and M.N. Cyrlin. 1985. The effect of blur upon static perimetric thresholds. *Doc Ophthal Proceedings Series* 42:563-567.

Caprioli, J., and G.L. Spaeth. 1985. Static thresholds examination of the peripheral nasal visual field in glaucoma. *Arch Ophthal* 103:1150-1154.

Drance, S.M. 1969. The early field defects in glaucoma. *Invest Ophthal* 8:84-91.

Drance, S.M., C. Wheeler, and M. Patullo. 1967. The use of static perimetry in the early detection of glaucoma. *Canad J Ophthal* 2:249-258.

Flammer, J., E. Eppler, and P. Niesel. 1982. Quantitative perimetry in the glaucoma patient without local visual field defects (in German). *Graefes Archiv* 219:92-94.

Flammer, J., G. Nagel, A. Glowazki, et al. 1981. Detection and definition of scotomata of the central visual field by computer methods. *Doc Ophthal Proceedings Series* 26:33-41.

Frisen, L. 1985. The earliest visual field defects in mid-chiasmal compression. *Doc Ophthal Proceedings Series* 42:191- 195.

Hard-Boberg, A., and J.D. Wirtschafter. 1985. Evaluating the usefulness in neuro-ophthalmology of visual field examination peripheral to 30 degrees. *Doc Ophthal Proceedings Series* 42:197-.206.

Hart, W. M., and B. Becker. 1977. Visual field changes in ocular hypertension. A computer based analysis. *Arch Ophthal* 95:1176- 1179.

Heijl, A. 1976. Automatic perimetry in glaucoma visual field screening. A clinical study. *Graefes Archiv* 200:21-37.

————. 1977. Time changes of contrast thresholds during automatic perimetry. *Acta Ophthal* 55:696-708.

————. 1983. Evaluation of automatic perimetry in glaucoma screening. In *Twenty-fourth International Congress of Ophthalmology, 1982,* Acta, ed. P. Henkind, Vol. 1, 162-165. Philadelphia: Lippincott.

————. 1985. The Humphrey Field Analyzer, construction and concepts. *Doc Ophthal Proceedings Series* 42:77-84.

Heijl, A., and S.M. Drance. 1980. Computerized profile perimetry in glaucoma. *Arch Ophthal* 98: 2199-2201.

Heijl, A., and C.E.T. Krakau. 1975. An automatic static perimeter, design and pilot study. *Acta Ophthal* 53:293-310.

Heijl A., and L. Lundqvist. 1983. The location of earliest glaucomatous visual field defects documented by automatic perimetry. *Doc Ophthal Proceedings Series* 35:153-158.

Heuer, D., M. Gressel, D. R. Anderson, et al. 1985. Does the Octopus Perimeter obey Weber's Law? *Invest Ophthal* 26(suppl):40.

Holmin, C., and C.E.T. Krakau. 1979. Variability of glaucomatous visual field defects in computerized perimetry. *Graefes Archiv* 210:235-250.

Katz, J. and A. Sommer. 1986. Automated threshold sensitivity among ocular hypertensives and controls. *Invest Ophthal* 27(suppl):44.

Keltner, J.L., and C. A. Johnson. 1981. Capabilities and limitations of automated suprathreshold static perimetry. *Doc Ophthal Proceedings Series* 26:49-55.

Klewin, K., and R. Radius. 1986. Background illumination and automated perimetry. *Arch Opthal* 104:395-397.

LeBlanc, R.P., and B. Becker. 1971. Peripheral nasal field defects. *Am J Ophthal* 72:415-419.

LeBlanc, R.P., A. Lee, and M. Baxter. 1985. Peripheral nasal field defects. *Doc Ophthal Proceedings Series* 42:377-381.

Leibowitz, H. M., et al. 1980. In *The Framingham eye study monograph. Surv Ophthal* 24(suppl):366-400.

Lynn, J.R. 1969. Examination of the visual field in glaucoma. *Invest Ophthal* 8:76-84.

Mikelberg, F.S., and S.M. Drance. 1984. The mode of progression of visual field defects in glaucoma. *Am J Ophthal* 98:443-445.

Mills, R. P. 1985. Usefulness of peripheral testing in automated screening perimetry. *Doc Ophthal Proceeding Series* 42:207-211.

Newman, S. A. 1987. Insensitivity of the automated monitoring system of the Octopus 2000R to small eye movements. *Invest Ophthal* 28(suppl):270.

*Perimetric Standards and Perimetric Glossary of the International Council of Ophthalmology.* 1979. ed. J.M. Enoch. The Hague: W. Junk.

Rock, W. J., S. M. Drance, and R. W. Morgan. 1971. A modification of the Armaly visual field screening technique for glaucoma. *Canad J Ophthal* 6:283-292.

————. 1973. Visual field screening in glaucoma. *Arch Ophthal* 89:287-290.

Sloan, L. 1961. Area and luminance of test object as variables in examination of the visual field by projection perimetry. *Vision Research* 1:121-138.

Werner, E. B., and S. M. Drance. 1977. Early visual
field disturbances in glaucoma. *Arch Ophthal*
95:1173-1175.

Wilensky, J.T., and B. C. Joondeph. 1984. Variation in
visual field measurements with an automated
perimeter. *Am J Ophthal* 97:328-331.

# Index